PRAISE FOR

TAI CHI—
THE PERFECT EXERCISE

"After my own decades of attempting to convey in ordinary English the deep and subtle insights of the Taoist traditions, I can appreciate the masterful contribution Arthur Rosenfeld had made with his *Tai Chi—The Perfect Exercise*. He brings sharp clarity to a subject too often shrouded in mystery and confusion."

—GUY LEEKLEY,
author of *Tao Te Ching:*
A New Version for All Seekers

"Whether you're a man or a woman, beauty starts from within. Trust Arthur Rosenfeld's easy-to-understand mind/body exercises to reduce your stress, increase your fitness, and transform you inside to out."

—PETER THOMAS ROTH,
CEO, Peter Thomas Roth Labs

"I have studied tai chi and qigong for thirty years, and found that all the most profound things I'd learned about these mind-body arts were not only represented in Arthur Rosenfeld's book *Tai Chi—The Perfect Exercise*, but profoundly articulated in a way that will benefit any teacher of any style. This book also successfully conveys the deeper and wider lessons tai chi and qigong offer as agents of compassionate change in a world hungry for such change, deftly using high science, chaos mathematics, and sociological facts and images to show how cutting edge and modern these ancient mind-body arts are. Thank you Arthur for this gift to tai chi and qigong and to the world."

—BILL DOUGLAS,
Founder of World Tai Chi & Qigong Day,
author of *The Complete Idiot's Guide to T'ai Chi & Qigong*

"Arthur Rosenfeld is one of the most special and genuine voices in the arts today. Not persuaded by fame, attention or self-congratulatory actions; he walks a path that is unique, winding and full of discoveries, surprises and truth, not just for himself but for those lucky enough to align themselves with him."

—DEL WESTON,
Martial Artist, Producer, Writer, and Director

"Rosenfeld's *Tai Chi* is as unique a contribution to the martial art as Bruce Lee's *Tao of Jeet Kune Do* was to his. This muscular work weaves history and modernity with philosophy and combat to create a tapestry that transcends all disciplines. Tai chi will travel with you regardless of where you go and regardless of whether you take it."

—CAMERON CONAWAY,
author of *Caged: Memoirs of a Cage-Fighting Poet*

"Arthur Rosenfeld is rightfully one of the foremost tai chi masters in this country if not the world. This mastery has spiraled into his writing. Although a Zen teacher, I have practiced tai chi for many years. This book has illumined my practice and offers fresh teaching examples in the areas of breath and energy that I can share with my students. I'm highly appreciative of his contribution with this work."

—MITCHELL DOSHIN CANTOR,
Sensei, The Southern Palm Zen Group

"Rosenfeld's book will improve your health and your mind. Easy and fun to read, it is filled with uplifting stories, lots to make you think about the world and plenty of easy-to-follow practical fitness advice. A delight."

—GRAEME MAXTON,
bestselling author and Fellow of the Club of Rome

"This book is not a 'how to' but rather a 'why you should'—an extended meditation on some of the central philosophical and physical tenets of tai chi as well as the physical and spiritual benefits the art can provide. Rosenfeld wisely uses his personal experience as a practitioner and his nuanced understanding of Taoist principles to explain how tai chi practice builds health and leads to an enhanced understanding of the human body. Each chapter explains significant aspects of tai chi physical principles, philosophy and ideas, finishing with exercises at three different levels that are designed to permit the reader to blend physical experience with conceptual insight....This a valuable and mature meditation on the virtually limitless depths of this art."

—JOHN DONOHUE,
author of the Connor Burke martial arts thrillers
Sensei, Deshi, Tengu and *Kage*

"Through stories, reflections and history lessons, Arthur Rosenfeld walks with us on a path that makes us question much of what we assume about exercise, health, values, and being. Tai chi is his theme, but his lessons are about living. You may find yourself looking for a local tai chi master when you are done, but you may also find yourself examining your life and your routines, inspired and empowered to make deep and healthy changes."

—STEPHEN ROSENFELD, M.D., M.B.A.,
Institutional Review Board Chair

TAI CHI

THE PERFECT EXERCISE

ALSO BY ARTHUR ROSENFELD

The Truth About Chronic Pain

TAI CHI
THE PERFECT EXERCISE

Finding Health,
Happiness,
Balance,
AND
Strength

ARTHUR ROSENFELD

Da Capo
LIFE
LONG

A Member of the Perseus Books Group

Photo Credits:
Page xii (Grand Master Chen Quanzhong and Master Max Yan) by Arthur
   Rosenfeld
All other photos by David Fryburg
Illustrations by Robin Ha

Printed in the United States of America.
For information, address Da Capo Press, 44 Farnsworth Street, 3rd Floor,
Boston, MA 02210.

Cataloging-in-Publication data for this book is available from the Library of
Congress.
First Da Capo Press edition 2013
ISBN: 978-0-7382-1660-7 (paperback)
ISBN: 978-0-7382-1661-4 (e-book)

Published by Da Capo Press
A Member of the Perseus Books Group
www.dacapopress.com

Note: The information in this book is true and complete to the best of our
knowledge. This book is intended only as an informative guide for those
wishing to know more about health issues. In no way is this book intended to
replace, countermand, or conflict with the advice given to you by your own
physician. The ultimate decision concerning care should be made between you
and your doctor. We strongly recommend you follow his or her advice.

Information in this book is general and is offered with no guarantees on the
part of the authors or Da Capo Press. The authors and publisher disclaim all
liability in connection with the use of this book.

Da Capo Press books are available at special discounts for bulk purchases
in the U.S. by corporations, institutions, and other organizations. For more
information, please contact the Special Markets Department at the Perseus
Books Group, 2300 Chestnut Street, Suite 200, Philadelphia, PA, 19103, or
call (800) 810-4145, ext. 5000, or e-mail special.markets@perseusbooks.com.

10 9 8 7 6 5 4 3 2 1

For all my teachers and all my students
past, present, and future.
Without you, I could not live the life I do and share the art I love.

"Though words cannot reveal the Source,
They do give meaning to the world we know."

TAO TE CHING (v. 1)
(Guy Leekley, Translator)

CONTENTS

ACKNOWLEDGMENTS

Master Max Yan deserves my biggest thanks for deepening my understanding of all the Taoist arts. His tai chi is simply without equal. Thanks also to Grandmaster Chen Quanzhong for setting the tone for my training. Over my protests, my illustrious agent, Bob Mecoy, who is always right, insisted I write this book. I'm glad I listened to him. My wonderful wife, Janelle, and my amazing son, Tasman, made the writing possible with their infinite forbearance—this work represents a shameful number of hours away from family activities. The flow and content here is thanks mostly to my editor, Renee Sedliar, without whom my ramblings would have been esoteric to the point of incomprehensibility. The look of the book owes much to David Fryburg's instinctive eye and magnificent photographs. Truly it would not be the visual treat it is without his contribution. Thanks to both my senior student, Jennifer Beimel, and my kung fu brother, Todd Plager, for their persistent proofing and suggestions. Thanks to Robin Ha for clean and clear illustrations, to Marco Pavia for helping it all come together, and to Jonathan Sainsbury and others at Da Capo who provided such a fine cover and balanced interior design.

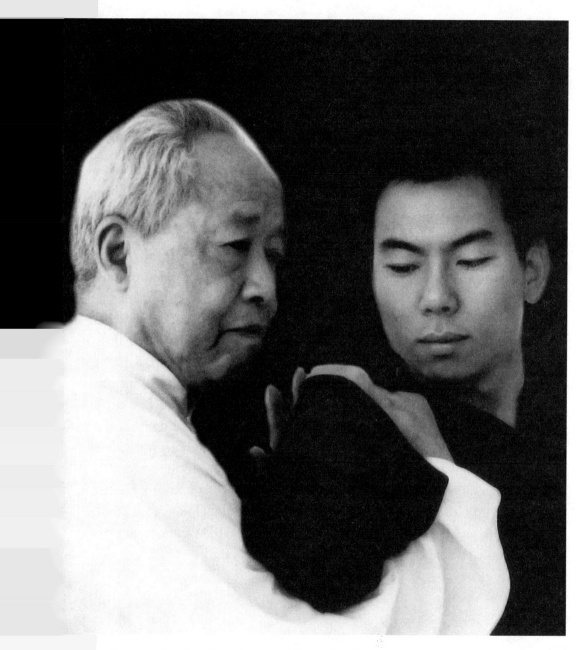

Grandmaster Chen Quanzhong and Master Max Yan

PREFACE

This book is a doorway into a world of physical magic and intellectual wonder. There is a great "stickiness" to the art of tai chi, a beguiling, pervasive quality that leads this quiet, wise, and introspective practice to seep inexorably into our consciousness. During the course of sustained practice, the borders between the old world we think we know and the new one we have just engaged grow increasingly blurred. Eventually, there is no border at all, and we are left with both a completely new way of looking at the way things work, and a new way to experience life.

Tai chi's pulsing, coherent, underlying intelligence fosters a sensitive and aware frame of mind, thus opening us to forces, trends, and patterns both inside our body and in the world around us. Practicing tai chi allows us to see and feel things differently on a physical, intellectual, emotional, and energetic level. It is the perfect art for the seeker—the person who has an abiding sense that contrary to the shallow, hurried model we're asked to embrace, there exists a deep, resource-rich alternative.

Growing up in New York City during the 1960s—a time in American history that was a veritable ballpark of ideas—I became such a seeker. Right from the start I found it very hard to believe and accept the values, priorities, and "facts" others took for granted. I was a weak kid, often sick and bedridden. Barred from the benefits of physical activities or sports—including the endorphin rush that makes exercise so pleasurable—I sought comfort in ideas that might help me better enjoy my world. Figuring that philosophers better understood what was really going on than anyone else, I engaged the works of Socrates, Plato, Russell, Buber, Sartre, Fromm (a family friend), and Hume, as well as Buddhist sutras, the Upanishads, the Bhagavad Gita, the Zen of D.T. Suzuki, and more.

Frequent intervals of illness were punctuated by intervals of cautious activity, but because I was overweight and chronically out of shape, gangs mugged me every few weeks on the streets of a far rougher New York City than the one that exists today. I had grown up keenly aware of unfairness and injustice, having lost a large chunk of my family to the Holocaust, and thus found both violence and threats of violence particularly difficult to tolerate. I began to entertain revenge fantasies, and gradually grew interested in the martial arts.

Film star Bruce Lee's philosophical aphorisms and David Carradine's contemplative rendering of a warrior monk in the television series *Kung Fu* suggested to me that martial training might help me create a better world for myself and those around me, and also help heal my body. Eventually I started to train and thereby became more confident and less fearful, more introspective and less extroverted.

During the ensuing thirty-three years I studied Western wrestling, Korean martial arts, Japanese fighting systems, American self-defense styles, Chinese performance disciplines, and finally, and exclusively, tai chi. That path shifted my focus from building strong muscles and good flexiblility to developing a sensitivity to the existence of energy and its flow—in martial arts terms from external to internal work.

I am privileged to enjoy a direct connection to the Chen family, which invented tai chi in the once-remote Chen family village, Chenjiagou, in Henan Province in the north of China. This connection evokes the ethos and ethics of the Hong Kong cinema from which

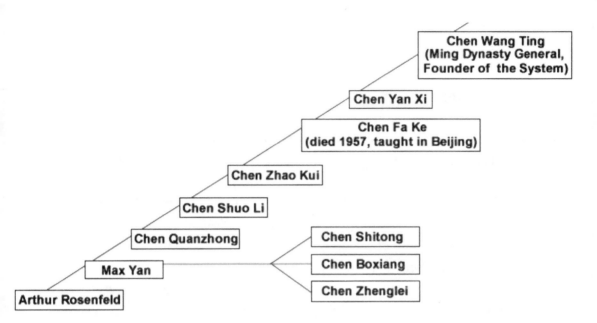

Bruce Lee took his production cues, for this is an art born of millennia of family tradition, of unimaginably rigorous and dedicated effort, of a connection to nature that bespeaks countless hours of silent observation spread over generations, centuries of battlefield testing, and the sacrifice of lives devoted to spiritual contemplation.

My secondary teachers are themselves members of the Chen family, while my primary teacher, Master Max Yan—a representative of a family so old it predates the formation of the nation we know as China—is an individual so brilliant and gifted he was trusted with knowledge by several Chen family masters. Some of these individuals were old enough to have used tai chi not only as a tool for self-cultivation and longevity, but also as a self-defense system in war. They were and are the keepers of family knowledge, writers, holders of the family archives, and devoted sages who have chosen to maintain a low profile in the face of tai chi's increasing visibility, popularity, and political vicissitudes. I am grateful to them for their humility, their high spiritual caliber, and for the marvelous and specialized information on tai chi energetics, application, weapons, and philosophy they have shared with me.

In addition to freeing me from the suffering and constraints endured by so many in our modern, materially obsessed and spiritually bereft climate, Master Yan showed me a way to heal my body and clear my mind while simultaneously teaching me much about the world and my place in it. He also helped me to grow and to heal in ways I had not dared to hope I could. Where I had been inflexible, I became supple; where I had been compromised, I flowered; where I had been delicate, I became robust; where I had been fearful, I became confident; where I had been quick to anger, I became patient; and where I had been overly consumed by my own welfare, I grew more and more compassionate and interested in the affairs of others. Over the years, tai chi has become my way of life.

What might this mean for you? Tai chi alters both the way we relate to people and the way we process events of our lives. Where once we saw differences if not opposition, we learn to see a nuanced, delicate interplay of opposing forces. Where once we saw only the surface of the pond of life, we become aware of constantly shifting, cyclical currents. Although tai chi requires no particular religious beliefs, practicing it can lead to a spiritual awakening, a sense of being part of a larger fabric of existence. As our inner life grows ever more luminous, the chatter of the speed-and-greed world slowly fades, leaving us with greater peace, tranquility, quiet, and contentment.

On a practical level, tai chi helps us to contend with the demands of career and family life with greater efficiency and poise. By simplifying the stories we tell ourselves about who we are and thereby getting in touch with our inner self, it helps us to better manage stress and anxiety and meet challenges more easily and without depletion. Unlike other physical activities, our tai chi tends to improve with age and time. Many older tai chi players (that is what we call each other) are able to perform feats that were out of reach when we were younger. Practicing tai chi, we age gracefully and with less drama, and we live longer, too.

Having been developed at a time when having trouble sitting still was neither an insult nor a symptom of some disorder, tai chi reveals to us the inalienable truth that our bodies were built to move, and that moving cures many of our ills. If sitting at a desk all day is the new smoking, then tai chi is the new yoga, offering us an opportunity to step out of contemporary culture's fast-moving river of modern life onto a stable, peaceful, natural island, a place where we can develop tranquility, relaxation, clarity, efficiency, and effectiveness. May this book serve as a bridge to that island.

HOW TO USE THIS BOOK

While *Tai Chi—The Perfect Exercise* is far from an encyclopedia and cannot hope to substitute for physical study with a qualified teacher, it does offer a range of content intended to serve both seasoned practitioners and those who are "interviewing" tai chi to see if it fits their transformational agenda. I have wherever possible avoided unnecessary reference to both ancient Chinese contexts and challenging terminology, instead addressing a range of concepts—from basic to advanced—in contemporary speech.

My first goal is to clearly explain how tai chi builds optimal health while facilitating a deep understanding of the workings of the human body. My second goal is to argue for tai chi's tremendous relevance in the modern world by showing how it deepens our understanding of the world and our place in it. Last but not least, I hope to clear up many myths and misunderstandings about the art, including some closely held by long-term practitioners.

Each chapter explores the movement, philosophy, and ideas specified in its title, and most provide exercises—termed "Explorations"—to deepen the understanding of the material offered. These Explorations draw on tai chi principles to lend insight into the practice and produce compelling benefits and results. They require no equipment save, in some places, small dumbbells. These explorations are not designed to teach tai chi, but rather issue a persuasive argument in favor of going out to find a teacher and class and then deepening and reinforcing what you have learned here with the help of your teacher. Presented in groups of three, each is more challenging than the previous so as to serve a range of age and fitness levels. It is best to start with the first exercise, practice it daily for a week or two, and then proceed to the next. Skipping an exercise, or even a day within your routine, means missing something: remember—tai chi is about the journey, not the destination.

Readers seeking tai chi's subtler dimensions, as well as practitioners already versed in the art, may wish to pay special attention to the sections labeled "Watercourse," a term from Chinese Taoist philosophy popularized by the mid-twentieth century philosopher Alan Watts, whose humorous and lucid explanations of Eastern concepts introduced to America a whole new way of seeing the world. All told I have presented a range of ideas that go beyond the details of the physical practice, hopefully providing plenty of "aha" moments along the way. The book is intended to be read as written, but jumping around throughout its pages can also be fun.

TAI CHI

THE PERFECT EXERCISE

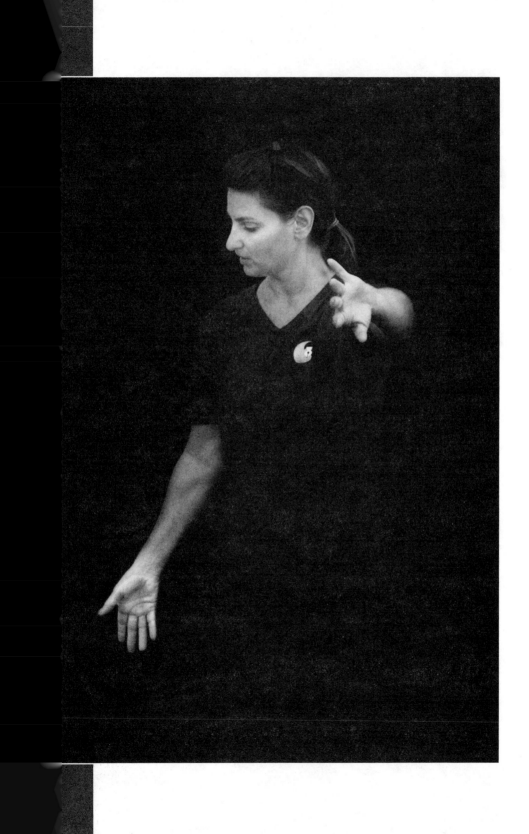

That martial arts are a system of self-defense is self-evident, and the medical benefits of martial exercise [are] not a great leap. However, Chinese culture has taken the martial arts several steps further, merging them with meditation and inner alchemy, and finally presenting them as a path of ultimate self-realization through the Tao.

DOUGLAS WILE, *LOST T'AI-CHI CLASSICS FROM THE LATE CH'ING DYNASTY*, 1996

INTRODUCTION—
WHAT IS TAI CHI?

Chances are good that you have seen tai chi in a neighborhood park. You may associate it with Asian people, pacifists, or aging hippies. You may also have heard that it is good rehab for heart patients and a fine way to manage stress. Perhaps you've been stirred by watching people practice tai chi with a sword, and inspired by how relaxed and precise they seem. You may even have seen tai chi on television, in Hong Kong kung fu movies and their recent Western derivatives such as *Crouching Tiger, Hidden Dragon* and *Kung Fu Panda*, or even in the cartoon series *Avatar: The Last Airbender*, which draws heavily on the art. Yet for all the impressions you may have, and all the curiosity, too, you likely cannot imagine the truly transformative potential of this marvelous art.

Long ago, tai chi was a system of battlefield fighting. Today, tai chi is a perfect exercise because it conditions the body, grows the spirit, and strengthens the mind. It is also a means of personal expression for millions of people around the world, an exotic paintbrush that can produce works of art as deep, rich, surprising, and rewarding as the people who wield it. Yet tai chi is more than an art form, a physical exercise, and a wondrous lens through which to see the world; it is a philosophy that can be lived, a lifestyle through which we can realize high ideals, and a complete recipe for health, longevity, happiness, and power.

Why is this so? How can something that appears to the untrained eye to be an exotic anachronism—a slow-moving physical irrelevance in a fast-paced virtual world—in fact represent a complex of ideas and body mechanics far, far greater and deeper than mere meditative dancing? How, when it is seen by most Westerners as something elderly people do in parks, can tai chi perform the miracles it does, from ameliorating arthritis pain to providing solace for the soul, from increasing core strength and enhancing balance to lending a mixed martial arts fighter a rapier eye for an opponent's weakness? How can such a superficially benign art enable the weak and small to overcome the strong and large while also opening a portal into the way the natural world works? The answer is that the set of concepts and techniques that comprise tai chi sit on a specific and remarkable tripod. The legs of the tripod are Taoist philosophy, the traditional martial arts of China, and Traditional Chinese Medicine (TCM).

TAOIST PHILOSOPHY

The Tao means the Way, and refers to an underlying force, intelligence, or cohering energy that pervades all that is. Taoism defines and dignifies us by virtue of our relationship with nature. To this day, many everyday folks, along with many priests, monks, and kung fu masters, attempt to follow the Tao, as do action heroes on both big and small screen, California surfers, Winnie-the-Pooh, and the film director/producer George Lucas, who, in his *Star Wars* movies, represented the Tao as "the force" and tai chi masters as Jedi knights.

Taoism recognizes cycles in all natural processes and appreciates the tension between opposites that makes our world what it is. These opposites are termed yin and yang. Examples include male and female, light and dark, up and down, Heaven and Earth, and rational and intuitive thought. When yin and yang are in proper balance—and unimpeded by certain typical qualities such as impatience, greed, impulsivity, self-centeredness, or self-delusion—a delightful, harmonious interplay occurs. The term for this interplay is tai chi, one that pertains to a philosophy and a lifestyle. The martial art that is the subject of this book is based on this harmonious exchange. The full and correct name of the art is actually tai chi ch'uan, where the word ch'uan means fist. This name denotes the fact that the most effective martial approach is to follow the natural balance of the universe.

In terms most relevant to tai chi, Taoism is expressed by a famous book presumed to have been written by Lao Tzu (an honorific that means Old Master) known as the *Tao Te Ching: The Classic of the Way and Virtue*. This short work discourses not only on the qualities of the superior man—the sage—but also upon the natural forces affecting our lives. The book suggests that the best way to hitch a ride on the running river of life is to be maximally effective with minimal effort. The Lao Tzu's early followers were woolly mountain men of the Middle Kingdom, Bacchanalian worshippers of nature who used herbs, meditation, and movement in pursuit of the Tao and in accordance with its rules. Such movements were closely related to the ones tai chi players now practice.

CHINESE MARTIAL ARTS

The tai chi tripod's second leg has a multi-thousand-year history of tried-and-true fighting techniques, whose interconnected influences have resulted in numerous beautiful martial arts styles. These are collectively known the world over—especially since the days of the film star, Bruce Lee—as "kung fu" or, more contemporaneously, wushu.

The phrase kung fu means hard and focused work, and can be applied to anything—from violin practice to chopping wood—to which a person dedicates time and effort. Martial kung fu is the province of warriors, for whom physical health and fitness has always been of paramount concern. It was never acceptable for someone who lives and dies by the sword to feel physically unprepared for combat on any given day or in any given situation. If maximum fitness was not available at every moment, the warrior risked a bloody death on the dusty road. In those days, the link between your mortality and taking the best possible care of yourself was abundantly clear. There was no debate about it, no conflicting social opinion trends, no magazines devoted to fitness and survival, no blog debates on efficacy or ethics, and no heated medical studies funded by companies selling health-related products.

Today, the link between exercise and health, while a topic of ever-growing interest, remains less immediate than it used to be. Health crises usually unfold much more slowly if no less dramatically than they did in the old days. Despite medical specialists, ambulances, and well-staffed emergency rooms, the death we risk in our modern society is often more protracted and prolonged than what an early warrior might suffer. Our modern healthcare system often allows us to survive abusing or neglecting ourselves. Still, if you seek self-actualization, personal fulfillment, and a long and happy life, being physically active is critical, and for some people self-defense skills can be a literal lifesaver.

Increasingly, kung fu training appeals to millions of people worldwide as a path to fitness and self-confidence. Unlike the many gym workouts primarily aimed at fashioning a beach or competition body, kung fu training emphasizes function over form. This is not to say "ripped" abs, "cut" arms, and "chiseled" buns cannot come from the training; rather, that the emphasis is on the way the body works more than on how the body looks. If you have in mind some old-style-kung-fu-movie-based notion of bells and buckets, bricks and ropes, rest assured that even in China, kung fu training has embraced all the modern tools and conveniences you find in any other fitness pursuit.

Some kung fu "styles" are named for the family that invented them, some for the regions from which they hail, some for their derivation from the movements of animals, and some for their association with legendary figures or mythic creatures. Regardless of their inspiration of geographic derivation, all are effective combat systems and rely more on sophisticated body mechanics and subtle body energies than on brute strength. These styles are broadly divided into northern Chinese and southern Chinese variants.

Northern styles show the influence of the famous Shaolin temple, and influences from Mongolia. Muslim fighting arts from what is now the Chinese province of Xinjiang are included in these battlefield systems, which feature the long-range weapons and long strikes born of conflict in wide-open spaces. Such arts prize strength, alignment, and connection to the ground, and are the source of their Japanese and Korean offspring, like karate and tae kwon do.

Southern styles of Chinese kung fu have a very different flavor. This part of East Asia is dominated by water, and where there is water, there are boats. Many formative-era conflicts occurred at close-quarters aboard ships, a platform for fighting that is by its nature unstable and restrictive. One cannot gallop with a lance in hand aboard ship, nor can one seek higher ground from which to dominate with devastating kicks. Southern fighting styles thus depend upon the opponent being at close range, and emphasize balance, stability, speed, and a keen sense of timing.

Tai chi belongs to a small, elite group of "internal arts" born of a mixture of the Northern and Southern attributes. Originally the province only of elite mercenaries and soldiers, it entails a program of physical training and the use of traditional Chinese weapons, and leads to superb physical and mental abilities. Internal arts emphasize softness over hardness, smooth movements, relaxation, sensitivity, and great control of balance, breath, and timing. The progression from so-called "hard or external" muscular training to soft, sensitive movements occurs within many Asian martial arts systems, but tai chi emphasizes relaxed softness from the outset. Such training is challenging and, even for the most athletically gifted person, requires time and practice. Thus, police officers who need to learn to subdue suspects quickly, soldiers about to ship out to an active war zone, or residents of dangerous urban environments might find tai chi very useful for stress control, but ought not choose it to make them martially effective in the shortest possible time.

Just because tai chi isn't quick and easy to learn, however, doesn't mean it has no self-defense value in the first few years of study. Setting aside the degenerative diseases of aging that become the greatest threat to most of us over time, it is also true that the solid, centered attitude that a tai chi person exudes deters opportunistic predators and bullies alike. More, a great number of violent encounters are forestalled before they occur simply by virtue of awareness and planning. To this tai chi brings the sort of clear, relaxed thinking that can help avoid a needlessly inflammatory response to a threat. In the long run, while bolstering your health, building your body, enhancing your longevity, and offering a lifetime of pleasure and satisfaction, tai chi can actually make you an excellent fighter. In the process, however, tai chi spiritual development will also teach you that violence is the lowest common denominator of human interaction.

TRADITIONAL CHINESE MEDICINE

Because tradition requires that a martial artist be able to heal the damage he or she inflicts, and because understanding the human body's intimate workings can lead to a useful martial understanding of its vulnerabilities, historically, many masters of the destructive arts were also capable healers. That is why the tai chi tripod needs its third leg, Traditional Chinese Medicine (TCM), a 5000-year-old system of prevention, diagnosis, treatment and cure. TCM's deep reservoirs include an intimate knowledge of indigenous herbs, a finely nuanced under-standing of the various cycles of fluid and substance in the body, and a familiarity with a term of subtle energy, called qi (pronounced "chee"), which Western scientists continue to study.

TCM's energy treatments, which manipulate qi using massage, acupressure, and acupuncture, are effective for both chronic and acute medical conditions. TCM's elaborate treatments for traumatic injury, which collectively fall under the name "bone setting," in some in-stances offer excellent alternatives to the standard of care in Western medicine, stimulating healing without surgical intervention, pinning, or the use of general anesthesia.

I have seen some amazing results from TCM, and these have flown in the face of the common perception that, while the system may be of some use for chronic conditions, it always pales in comparison to the miracles of modern Western medical technology in treating acute con-ditions. This view may not be the complete story. If I were hit by a bus, I would indeed prefer the life-saving techniques of Western trauma medicine to reattach my leg, stuff my viscera back where it belongs, and keep my heart pumping through it all. After that, though, I might well opt for an integrated approach that includes TCM.

My father, the world-famous cardiologist Dr. Isadore Rosenfeld, visited China in the 1970s and witnessed open-heart surgery con-ducted with only acupuncture anesthesia, the patient awake and talk-ing as the procedure was performed. His account of what he saw, published in *Parade Magazine*, created a small firestorm of contro-versy, in part because at that time, more so than today, acupuncture and other forms of TCM were perceived as voodoo medicine.

It certainly isn't voodoo. As my research for my documentary films substantiates, there is much that is real and effective about TCM, acupuncture included. Some years ago a physician and fellow tai chi player and I were visiting a bonesetter in Bamboo County, Guangdong Province, China. Bonesetters in China approximate chiropractors in the West, with a good dose of osteopathy thrown in. This particular master of the art was born to a bonesetting family know for its techniques, skills, and secrets. While I was visiting his clinic, a teenage boy was brought in fresh from a motorbike accident. He had a complex fracture of his arm, with many breaks and bones fragments out of line. Here in the West, repairing this complex injury would have required general anesthesia, surgery, and the insertion of pins.

Such advanced options are not often available in rural China. Instead, I saw the bonesetter begin his treatment by inserting a couple of needles in the injured arm. Instantly, the boy, who had been white from pain and clammy from shock was able to relax and smile. After that, the bonesetter put his hands on the arm, closed his eyes, and with great concentration began to literally reassemble the arm, gently lining up the major bones and guiding the fragments back into place on the basis of touch alone. He then wrapped the arm in something akin to cheesecloth and applied a poultice of herbs that hardened in place, creating a light cast. "Leave it on for a week," he told the boy, "then come back and we will put on another one, with different healing herbs." When he was finished, he took an x-ray to show my doctor friend, who studied the image carefully. "We couldn't do this at home," my friend said. "It puts us to shame."

BENEFITS IN A NUTSHELL

Having defined tai chi as a coalescence of philosophy, self-defense, and medicine, it's easy to imagine the art's benefits falling into related categories, and they do. Looking first at the health benefits, it's easy to be incredulous. Indeed, The Harvard Women's Health Watch says of tai chi, "This gentle form of exercise can prevent or ease many ills of aging and could be the perfect activity for the rest of your life."[1]

There is now so much evidence that the practice lowers blood pressure, aids in sleep, increases the immune response, improves flexibility and balance, strengthens the body's core muscle groups, improves focus and concentration, and is of benefit in easing a variety of disease states including asthma, insomnia, arthritis, chronic fatigue, Parkinson's, hypertension, and more. There is even work underway to document how tai chi alters the structure of our DNA! Impressive though these data may be, they merely hint at what tai chi can do for you, in part because there is always more investigating to do, and in part because that bedrock of Western medicine—the double blind, placebo-controlled study—has limitations when it comes to tai chi. That's due to the fact that such studies require an investigator to be able to identify and isolate variables that, in the case of tai chi, remain elusive and poorly defined. In short, it is difficult to find something when you know neither where or what it is.

Scrutinizing tai chi's benefits through the lens of Western medicine may actually lead us to miss the forest for the trees. That's because of Western science's fondness for deconstructing things into their component parts so as to understand them on the one hand, and TCM's penchant for thinking in terms of relationships and systems on the other. In Western terms, we can say that unlike more common exercises such as tennis, football, baseball, jogging, golf, swimming, or cycling, tai chi is a mind/body practice of the sort that yoga is intended to be, offering benefits that transcend the purely physical. Intellectually understanding tai chi's philosophical concepts leads to a change of mind, and performing tai chi movements leads to a change of body. When the mind and body engage in a dialogue of hormones and neurotransmitters, the transformational effects of the practice are enhanced in an exponential way. In TCM terms, we can say that as a system, tai chi benefits the level and distribution of our energy by bolstering some dimension of movement here, some emotional and intellectual facet there.

In a very real sense, tai chi is a laboratory for the comprehension of Taoist principles, a refuge from the fray of life wherein to test one's understanding of balance, harmony, sensitivity and power. Such testing leads to growing of the inner self rather than cultivating a focus on external trappings, with the result that the world of emotions and sensations becomes more interesting than the external material frenzy of the modern world. The first step toward this reorienting is the removal of all unnecessary muscular tension from the body. This is a profound enterprise, because daily stress—a common manifestation of inappropriate tension—is well known to be the source of more doctor visits than any other single factor.

The second step in changing how we move through the world is to become more efficient and thereby tire less easily and accomplish more in everything we do throughout the day. Moving in this new way, our muscles grow stronger, our brain masters new patterns of perception and action, and our joints open in response to the spiraling energy patterns that are unique to tai chi. This overall process begins with the very first tai chi class and intensifies exponentially until the art takes up residence in our meat and bone.

The third step in transforming ourselves with tai chi is to achieve a harmonious mental state, which means learning to be keenly aware of our own emotions and to consistently take a deeper and more philosophical view of challenges. We come to nip negative thoughts and feelings in the bud and healthfully channel irrational exuberance. Rather than succumbing to the sticky pull of other people's problems, tai chi people navigate relationships relatively unencumbered by worry, lack of self-confidence, and misapprehension. The resulting cool balance is termed wuji (pronounced "woo-jee") and is one of the great goals and benefits of tai chi practice. The wuji mind deepens our vision, allows us to clearly see exactly what needs to be done, and specifically equips us to find creative solutions to conflict. In situations where one option, or door, is to meet force with force and a second door is to yield and be overrun, the wuji mind is often able to find a third door that represents a unique solution acceptable to both parties. Because such creative clarity often leads to compassionate action, people who do not study tai chi might term the third door a random act of kindness when it is more accurately a deliberate act of consciousness.

As a fourth benefit, tai chi builds physical energy. Physical work now seems less daunting to the tai chi person, who discovers a reservoir of strength that allows him/her to endure and prevail in many different situations. The particular fashion in which tai chi builds energy also harmonizes the interaction between the body's organ systems, allowing them (according to the TCM model) to enhance sexual essence. Many people are drawn to Taoist exercises out of desire to increase their sexual enjoyment and performance, and they find that tai chi does wonders for their sex life.

SO WHAT DOES TAI CHI LOOK LIKE?

Tai chi practice typically consists of a series of movements brought together like pearls on a string. Some people call the movements "postures," an unfortunate word because a posture is static and tai chi is dynamic; without movement, tai chi does not exist. Taken together, the movements of tai chi are referred to as a "form." Some tai chi forms are performed slowly, others are quite quickly and vigorously. Performing tai chi feels simultaneously relaxing and powerful. It leaves the player with the sense that she is moving in accordance with human structure and the laws of gravity, leverage, and inertia. Whether done dreamily and slowly or quickly with martial intent, tai chi embodies strong grace.

Tai chi is as much a state of mind as it is a system of movement. Demanding presence and attention to every sensation and detail, tai chi flees the moment the mind wanders. The instant we think about the pizza we're planning to have for lunch, worry about whether the babysitter is into the wet bar, glance at the sky to track an impending thunderstorm, feel a chill in our spine about an upcoming exam or performance review, tai chi in its pure sense goes out the window. Let the mind slip away to an interlude with a lover, pop off to a happy memory of a tropical vacation or the best margarita we've ever tasted, and because tai chi is all about the mind/body connection, it's gone.

Return to awareness of the present moment, feel our muscles, our connective tissue, our joints and our bones, and tai chi returns. Because it requires a completely inwardly directed consciousness, genuine tai chi is not a performance and should not be done with an audience in mind.

Geometricians and physicists know that the spiral is nature's archetypal shape, being found in galaxies, tornadoes, seashells, the flow of liquid through pipes (or blood vessels) and water exiting a drain. In recognition of this natural design, tai chi movements—particularly Chen style, the founding family's original art—characteristically describe spirals. Spiral movement is a sign of tai chi's Taoist origins, and accounts for the fact that many people watching tai chi say that in addition to looking exotic and graceful, the practice also appears organic and natural

Natural, however, does not mean easy. While tai chi is adaptable to fitness levels from wheelchair-bound patients to Olympic athletes and suitable from ages 12 to 112, the art challenges us at every level. Every student soon becomes aware that every movement has onion-like layers of depth and complexity. Watching tai chi in a local park, health club, senior center, or martial arts school, it will immediately become apparent—even within a single class—which players have been at it the longest. A seasoned tai chi practitioner usually exhibits smoother movements, seems more relaxed, may sink lower in his stances, and may perform strikes with percussive authority.

The original purpose of form practice was to test martial strength and alignment and to remain strong, rooted (more on this later), and relaxed in the kind of unpredictable situations a real-life battle might bring. In the battlefield of everyday life today, and with a focus on health and longevity, these beautiful movements function to enhance our balance, sensitivity, serenity, composure, and power. While the elderly and infirm player can find plenty of benefit in performing tai chi gently and in a high stance, the fittest, strongest, most flexible athlete can crouch on one leg or go into deep and challenging stances. Form practice coordinates upper and lower extremities at every athletic level, all the while strengthening the body right down to the marrow.

As the tai chi onion suggests, traditional tai chi training follows a set curriculum. Each grade, or level, requires you to be able to do certain things. At the beginning, the focus is on relaxing the upper body, shifting the weight properly, and learning arm circles and stances. As the student's skill grows, the requirements become more demanding, traditional Chinese weapons such as straight and curved swords, spear, halberd, sticks, mace, and the long pole may be brought into play to build strength, increase mobility, sensitivity, and flexibility, and improve footwork and timing. Simplified tai chi will not include such tools, but if you find an advanced group at a park or martial arts school you may be lucky enough to catch a glimpse of the art's martial roots.

BUT IS IT THE RIGHT CHOICE?

It is if we like the idea of developing our body and mind together. It is if we cherish function as much as form and love a strong muscular core. It is if we want sculpted thighs and a great rear end. It is if we want the toned upper body advanced tai chi training with partners and traditional weapons provides. It is if extreme forms of fitness training don't appeal (yet real power does), and if we take a long-term view of health. It is if we've always hated the gym but love to exercise outside. It is the right choice if we fancy a discipline that can be done competitively or as a deeply personal journey, wherever fate or fortune may take us, no matter our age, fitness level, or strength. It is the right choice if we find joy in learning about ourselves over time.

Tai chi is a good fit for us if we have the discipline to stay the course even when the training is difficult, trusting that there must be a reason why it has benefited millions of people for hundreds of years. It is a good fit if we have always been seekers, both for deeper ways of understanding the way the world works and for a better appreciation for how to use our body in sophisticated new ways we may not even be able to imagine right now. Certainly, tai chi is a good fit if we are always rushing around and wish, just for a few hours at least, that we could slow down and have time to more deeply experience life's intricacies, opportunities, and pleasures.

In the northern Chinese village where tai chi was invented, the art is taught to young children and enjoyed throughout all stages of life. In fact, in the many years I have taught and practiced, I have seen many students bust stereotypes regarding who is best suited to the art. It turns out that there is not much correlation at all between success in tai chi and advancing years, nor with youth and vigor, great athletic aptitude, coordination, stamina, flexibility, or strength. Tai chi develops all these qualities, but they are not required for a seat at the tai chi table. Indeed, neither is being Chinese, or having an intense interest in pugilism or Asian martial arts. Being a dancer, a cyclist, ball player, or swimmer yields no particular tai chi advantage, nor does proficiency at yoga.

The best predictor of future success in the art is the ability to embrace bewilderment. The first weeks and months of tai chi class can be a struggle for the kind of person who feels compelled to understand every detail of what they are doing. We must be able to practice movements over and over, trusting that in time they will reveal their riches. In addition to swallowing doubts, it helps not to measure our progress against that of our classmates or against some imagined standard; there is little relationship between how quickly we master the exterior pattern of a movement and how competent a tai chi player we ultimately become.

Our love affair with tai chi—yes, over time many people do fall in love with the art—will carry us through those early classes where we are simultaneously lost in Chinese names and bedazzled by the grace and fluidity of a teacher's moves. Tai chi teaches us that life is not all about merely getting things done; we all know how it ends, so rushing through life is just senseless. If tai chi sounds like a long-term investment, that's because it is. The good news, however, is that the required commitment arises organically as it does in any relationship that is worth the time and effort. The art reminds us not to rush from one activity, project, or relationship to the next, as in the large sense all human endeavors are the same. It teaches us to be here now and treasure the journey over the destination. The art may even shake our inappropriate preoccupation with outcome and achievement, a fresh shift for many Westerners.

Tai chi is the right choice if the quiet intricacy and elegance we see when we watch a class appeals to us, if we feel the draw of an ancient, deep, exotic practice. It is the right choice if we want to connect to the world in new ways, and if we need new methods ways of handling stress and conflict. It is a good fit for us if we want to build mindfulness and purer attention, and if belonging to a community of people who are more spiritual than material sounds nurturing. In the end, tai chi is for us if we believe that anything worth doing is worth doing slowly.

Effort and Effortlessness

In his *Tao Te Ching*, Lao Tzu says, "The sage does nothing, but somehow gets everything done." With this phrase, he is trying to explain that his easy, natural way is the best route to accomplishing things—a freeway of sorts—even though most people would rather exhaust themselves climbing a steep mountain path because they believe that if no effort is required, the goal is unworthy. It is amazing how what was true thousands of years ago in China is true in America today; the notion that suffering and perseverance is somehow validating persists.

The relevance to tai chi practice should be clear. Nothing gets results faster than following the body's natural cadence and rhythm. There is no better way to make progress in the art than to become mindfully sensitive to the cues coming from our body, and responding to those cues with methodical practice. Pushing to the point of great soreness slows us down. Balancing the forces at work within and without our body is the straightest and fastest route to tai chi proficiency, even though we have been trained to think that pushing like a Navy Seal, lifting like a bodybuilder, and enduring pain stoically are signs of character.

This means that practicing moderately and consistently brings better results than training episodically but with extreme gusto. Concentrating on the quality of our relaxation, sinking, and turning is a better strategy than worrying about how many hours we put in. In tai chi we must remember that straining to overcome an opponent means we are doing something wrong. Rather than relying on muscular force we should rely on sensitivity and skill. Success should surprise us when it comes. Try too hard, force things along, and you are in the mountains when you should be on the straight, direct road. Tai chi is all about efficiency, effectiveness, and effortless action.

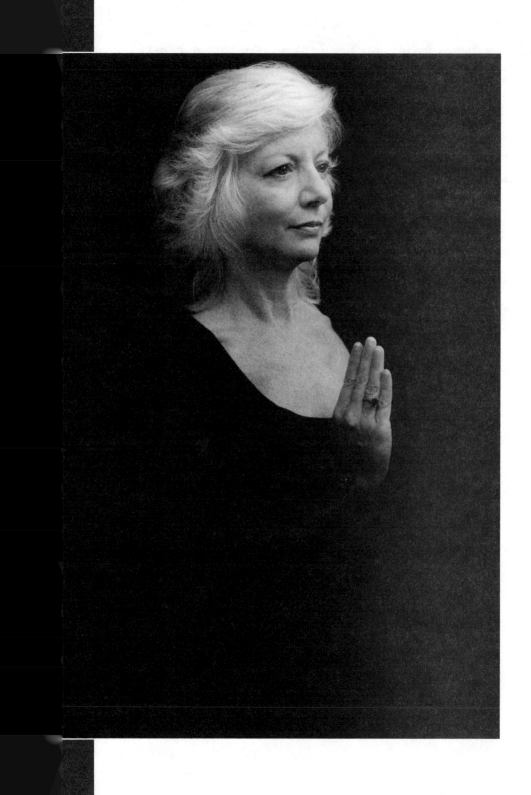

The soft and weak
overcome the hard and strong.
TAO TE CHING, V.36 (HOLLY ROBERTS, TRANSLATOR)

RELAXING INTO THE WORLD

Consumer culture, relentlessly negative media messages, and the unsustainable depletion of natural resources combine to make healthy choices hard to find. Sometimes we accept harmful lifestyle influences because we believe we have no choice; sometimes we unwittingly make choices that seem right at the time but are not in our long-term physical or spiritual best interest. We may, for example, deny ourselves sleep in favor of working to make money to buy things we don't need. Too, we may ignore a pain in our chest because we're more afraid of the cost of care than we are about our health.

Although we are biologically adaptable enough to live by the seacoast, near a lake, in a forest, a city, or at altitude, we are also often prone to preoccupations and delusions that lead us to deny our spiritual, emotional, and physical needs. When we do this, we experience stress, which makes us tense and anxious. Our joints start to ache, our sleep and digestion suffer, and we may even become depressed. Tai chi is so effective at countering a multitude of stressful and unhealthy influences because it is built on the tripod discussed in the introduction—practical kung fu, Traditional Chinese Medicine, and Taoist philosophy. These elements are present at every level of the practice, from a single move to an entire training program.

When a system maintains its design elements at every level from the minutest detail to the most elaborate technique, we call it a fractal. To better understand the concept, let's consider the pyramid at Giza. If that famous monument were a fractal (it isn't), then if we drove a bulldozer into it, the boulders that broke off would all be shaped exactly like small pyramids. If we took a sledgehammer to those boulders, they would break into pieces that were even smaller pyramids. If we pulverized those small pyramids into dust and looked at them under a microscope, we would see tiny pyramids akin to the Giza giant in every aspect from density to proportion.

Our universe is full of fractals. It could be said, for example, that on the grandest scale, galaxies express the overall order of the universe, and are, in turn, fractally represented on a smaller scale by solar systems. Planets fractally represent the solar systems to which they belong. Many creatures living on earth are fractals of the planet that supports them, having skeletons, blood vessels, and moods in much the way the earth has continents, rivers, and weather.

Because tai chi is a fractal, every time we practice—indeed every time we perform even a single tai chi move—we bring the principles, shape, intelligence, and architecture of the whole system to bear on the goal of transforming our bodies and our lives. The very principle, and in some ways the most important lesson we learn from tai chi, is how to relax. When we are relaxed, we are less likely to be influenced by harmful forces that can poison the way we look at the world and our place in it. Free of such influences, we understand more clearly how to change the way we use our bodies and beneficially interact with our environment.

THE IRON LOLLIPOP

Conjure if you will the classic U.S. Marine Corps recruiting poster of yore, the one bearing the tagline "the few, the proud, the Marines." In this presentation of America's fighting finest, a row of men stands in dress uniform, rifles tucked in beside them, carrying themselves beautifully, with chests jutting and eyes forward. This straight posture is the archetypal one not only for a strong man, but for a graceful woman as well. The trouble is that while ballerinas manage their erect carriage by specifically training the muscles it requires, career soldiers—guards standing duty at an embassy post come to mind—may exaggerate their positions and rely on iron discipline to force their body up and forward. The result is that career military men often complain of inflexible torsos, low back pain, tender and restricted shoulders, hypertension, and more.

Holding too much stiffness in our body, we are like a lollipop that has turned from candy to iron. Top heavy and tense, we stress our heart, ruin our balance, and create musculoskeletal problems. Tai chi helps us to slide that iron lollipop down the stick, lowering our center of gravity, making us more stable and relaxed. The more relaxed we become, the more sensitive we are to environmental inputs ranging from pheromones, facial expressions, aromas, threatening body language, changes in temperature, nighttime sounds that are out of the ordinary, and a thousand other energetic harbingers of danger, opportunity, and more.

Without tension and with the lollipop low down, our body hangs as effortlessly as the skeleton in our high school science room. Imagining a string connecting the top of our head with heaven, we cultivate a nice, upright posture and forward gaze without effort. We focus on dropping and releasing every part of us right down to the molecular level, feeling the tension depart as we lower our center of gravity along our spine from the top of our head to the midpoint of our perineum.

SPECIFICS OF TAI CHI RELAXATION

Tai chi relaxation is a very particular phenomenon. It has nothing to do with kicking back on the family room couch with a beer in one hand and the television remote in the other. The Chinese term for tai chi relaxation is *fan song*, and it connotes linking mind and body in such a way that great internal and external awareness combine to allow us to unwind. Rather than lying on the ground as in a yoga corpse pose, tai chi relaxation takes place within a structured context. Tai chi players release tension in the muscles of the neck, back, and hips while building strength in the muscular core—particularly gluteal and abdominal groups—along with the thigh muscles (quadriceps).

One way to envision tai chi relaxation in a physical sense is to imagine that your torso is an egg and your pelvis is like a porcelain cup used to serve poached eggs in the old days. Our head is the top of the egg and points up, while the larger, rounded end of the egg is your lower belly and sits down into the circumference of the cup, our pelvic girdle. Settling the torso into the pelvis while keeping the spine straight (no leaning front to back or side to side) results in an even, downward force. This force widens and deepens the pelvic area and helps to loosen and open our hips. Open, relaxed hips are required to perform most tai chi movements properly.

The tai chi player quickly notices that *fan song* causes a burn in the thigh muscles, a sign we are on the right track both to greater relaxation and to stronger legs. Imagine the two variables, leg strength and degree of fan song sitting on opposite ends of a seesaw. As we relax more, the relaxation side of the seesaw goes down. In response to the workout, our muscles grow, we get stronger, and the leg strength end of the seesaw goes down. This process continues, with strength and relaxation alternating and stimulating each other, as our tai chi ability increases.

The binary way in which strength and relaxation interrelate evokes the classic yin/yang symbol, technically the symbol for tai chi. In that symbol the white half of the circle has a black dot in it and the black half has a white dot. In the context of tai chi body mechanics, this suggests that relaxation has a bit of strength in it and strength a bit of relaxation. The overall circular shape of the symbol, moreover, suggests that the relationship is turning, moving, continuous, and supported by our mind. In Western medical terms, we could say that in response to cues from the body, the brain calms down, leading to feelings of well-being, emotional stability, and satisfaction. In turn, our our muscles surrender their tension—and organs and viscera function more healthfully—in response to cues from our mind.

In the framework of Traditional Chinese Medicine, relaxation and proper alignment facilitate the flow of our vital energy, qi. Qi must flow in unrestricted fashion—and must be present in ample quantity and correct quality—for us to be optimally healthy. As a garden sprinkler system nourishes our plants and grass, so our qi nourishes our organs, muscles, viscera, bone, and brain. In the same way a bare patch or wilting bush suggests a corrupted pipe, various medical problems indicate that our qi flow has been adversely affected. As a break, bend, or clog can reduce the flow of water through a pipe, so stress, tension, poor posture, or incorrect movement adversely affects the flow of qi through our meridians.

These are just different ways of understanding how tai chi relaxation not only leads to suppleness, power, and youthful energy, but to a clear mind that communicates in unfettered fashion with the body and with the people and situations it encounters. It may seem counterintuitive that a relaxed hand, a hand held almost loose, can express more power than an overly tight fist. It may seem even more unlikely that a body moving as loose as an orangutan's can deliver more power than "Iron" Mike Tyson's nastiest roundhouse. Yet orangutans, gorillas, and human babies—incredible powerhouses all—intuitively know that to be at their strongest, they have to commit their whole body to each and every movement in relaxed and focused fashion, and do so with their "pipes" patent and qi flowing.

HARMONIOUS BODY MECHANICS

The black-and-white tai chi symbol also describes how our muscles, working in opposing groups called flexors and extensors, rely upon each other for ideal function; when one tightens, the other loosens. Think of executing a straight punch. Muscles on the backside of our arm, such as the triceps brachii, work to extend the arm at the shoulder and elbow joints, while muscles on the front side, including the biceps brachii, must release. Ideally, the extensors work without even a tiny bit of opposition from the contractor muscle groups. The pain of stubbing a toe or jamming a finger reminds us of the power inherent in such unfettered, natural movement. As infants, we always move this way; as we get older, the stresses of civilization take their toll and we often move tensely and against our own purpose. Tai chi trains us to return to pure, relaxed movement. Part of this training is technique, part of it is relaxation, and part of it involves adopting new ideas.

One such idea is "the Three External Harmonies," a kung fu concept that describes cooperative body movement. The first of three external harmonies reminds us that the shoulders should be aligned with the hips for balance and for the proper delivery of force. This means that we should be able to draw a line from the middle of the shoulders to the middle of the hips and see some congruence there. If the body is twisted or the shoulders are off to one side (note that this does not mean one cannot bend, just that the torso and lower body must remain lined up) force will not be transmitted properly. It also suggests that shoulder movement must originate in the hips. This is a helpful reminder that many of us carry a great deal of stress and tension in the shoulders, sometimes as a result of too much computer work and sometimes from the "I carry the world on my shoulders" syndrome.

The second of the Three External Harmonies defines the relationship between the elbows and the knees. When the elbows are closer to each other (in tight to the body), an opponent has little leverage on us and our balance is not vulnerable. Therefore we can assume a narrow stance, which is riskier in terms of balance but more agile, allowing us to move in and out of a position faster. Conversely, when our arms are extended and our elbows far apart, our opponent can find a lever to use against us easily, so our knees must be far apart to create a stance that is slow to enter and exit but is wide and stable.

The last of the Three External Harmonies relates the wrists and ankles—or, as some teachers put it, the feet and the hands—conveying the idea that we should always be aware of how our weight distribution affects the power in our hands. Biomechanically speaking, when we strike, grab, parry, or lock, the power to our hand most often comes from the ground under our opposite foot. The accomplished tai chi player dances with gravity, offering the opponent as a "tribute" to gravity so long as the player himself is allowed to remain standing.

Tai chi's mind/body dimension suggests that the Three External Harmonies be augmented and balanced by Three Internal Harmonies, and indeed they are. The first of these speaks to the relationship between our emotional state, *xin*, and our martial intention, *yi*. Simply put, this tells us we have to believe in what we're doing if we are to control our fear and act. Fear for our own life—"stay away from me!"—or concern for another—"I won't let you hit that kid again!"— stirs our *xin* and focuses our *yi* to galvanize us into action.

The second internal harmony connects our yi to our life force, qi, as a general commands his troops. Imagine that the general has a military objective that is on the other side of a narrow ravine. Archers line the ridge on each side of the top of the ravine, their bows aimed down at the general's forces. Seeing the situation, the troops request an audience with the general and tell him that if they launch a direct, frontal assault the archers will wipe them out. A poor general will ignore his men and send them in anyway, figuring that maybe a few will get through. In life, as in tai chi, this means planning without paying attention to circumstances or physical limitations.

A better kind of general, the kind of *yi* that we want in our tai chi practice, listens courteously to his troops and then cooperatively devises a strategy to both preserve his force and accomplish his objective.

Perhaps, for example, he breaks his forces into four parts, sending two flanking expeditions to climb the ridge and take out the archers, while a third makes a feint for the belly of the ravine, and defended by shields, draws fire. When the arrows are expended and the ridgeline archers removed, the main, real fighting force can go through. That's the kind of dialog this second internal harmony suggests occur between our intention and our life force, and one that pervades tai chi practice.

The third internal harmony pertains to the relationship between our *qi* and our strength, or *li*. *Qi* supplies the "juice" to perform a task, whereas muscles provide *li*. Tai chi requires us to be soft and relaxed but it also requires us to be physically strong. Considering all six harmonies now, three external and three internal, we can see how the system depends upon a relaxed mind and body to go all the way from emotion to result, using energy and good body mechanics along the way.

REJUVENATION AND REPAIR

Focusing solely on results is fine while rescuing buried earthquake victims or searching for a cure for cancer, but may not be the best approach when trying to enhance health, longevity, spiritual depth, and emotional satisfaction. The tai chi path—constantly changing, evolving, shifting, always flexible and never rigid—is more a watercourse than it is a mountain trail, and is most emphatically a journey not a destination. Tai chi deepens our ability to process information and allows us to identify new options. Those options, in turn, often result in a change of goals. It is true that tai chi form practice can help our golf game and tai chi sensitivity drills can enhance our sex life, but a single-minded fix on goals closes us to additional opportunities we may not have even realized were possible when we set those goals. Tai chi turns back our clock to the time when our life's possibilities were endless, our needs were clear, our intentions obvious, our body supple, our movements pure and quick, and our results more or less assured.

In childhood, when we were relaxed and receptive, we were open to anything and everything.

If we allow it to do so, our tai chi practice can bring us back to that state—and in the process repair much of the damage we have sustained in the interim. Part and parcel of such allowing is to surrender to the art and have it suffuse and motivate us, creating both revelations and new syntheses between our beliefs, attitudes, perceptions, and actions. Rather than using the art as we might a sport or piece of equipment (with the intention, say, of becoming more fit) tai chi uses us to express its principles in the world. Surrendering to this process requires self-confidence, discipline, dedication, and trust both in the good intentions of our teacher and the wisdom of the masters behind her.

Body workers such as chiropractors, massage therapists, and acupuncturists know that long-term structural and physiological problems acquire an emotional dimension and are therefore more challenging to address than recent injuries. That's why mind/body practices are so helpful for these chronic issues. Tai chi, a favorite prescription among many healthcare professionals, provides a laboratory in which we can investigate the treasured tango between body and mind. Exploring the link between our emotional experience and movement, we may at first struggle to accept that what we feel physically has anything to do with our emotions. The more we relax, however, the more we give certain realizations permission to rise to the conscious level. For example, we may come to realize that our poor posture is the result of having long ago been judged, castigated, or hit. We may discover that we hold tension in our jaw, neck, shoulders, or hips because both sleep and free time were in short supply during childhood.

Revelations about the mind/body relationship require quiet practice time into which we can unfold and expand. Unfortunately, modern culture leads to behaviors like consuming, hurrying, and judging, that drive us to distraction, not introspection. Tai chi balances these lifestyle problems by revealing our true nature to us, stripped of the physical and emotional clutter that—just like a garage full of "stuff"—later accrue.

Steadfast practice can actually lead to more than just realization of the emotional root of our physical discomfort and limitation. It can also lead to an actual shift in our life paradigm. While stripping away what we've suffered in order to get back to a simpler, healthier, happier us, we may also find ourselves coming to trust the Tao—the nature of things—and in doing so embrace a completely new way of engaging work, relationships, dreams, and desires. On a more material and mundane level we may find that tai chi body mechanics help us accomplish everyday tasks such as washing dishes or mowing the lawn, and we may learn to match the daily peaks and valleys of our life energy, our qi, so as to become more effective and efficient. Tai chi balances our yin and our yang and allows us to relax into life.

EXPLORATION #1

Tensing and Relaxing

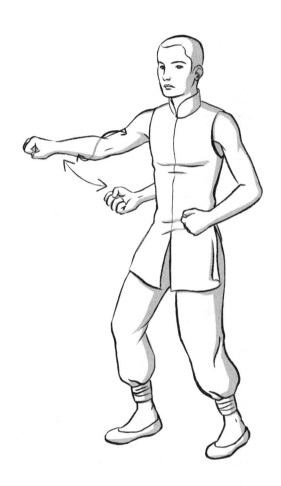

THIS FIRST EXERCISE TEACHES YOU TO QUICKLY AND EASILY let go of muscular tension. It's a good stress management tool and a fun way to introduce tai chi magic into your life. Begin by standing with your feet shoulder-width apart, then lower your body as if sitting down into a bar stool or tall chair. As you drop, ease back into your hips to create an inguinal crease (a fold where the leg and torso meet), not going so far that your toes lift and lose balance. Keeping your body as perfectly straight as possible, sink gradually, bending your knees less than the angle of your inguinal crease. If you are fit and strong and accustomed to bending deeply you may continue sinking until your thighs are parallel to the ground, the knee is at a right angle, and the lower leg creates a straight column down to the ground.

Starting with your hands by your waist, slowly extend the right fist in a punching motion while simultaneously inhaling and tensing every muscle from the head to foot. Grabbing the ground with your toes, activate the calf muscles, squeezing the buttocks and belly, stiffening the chest, shoulders, and neck, tense the upper and lower back, too. The punch should take about five seconds. Once your fist is fully extended with the elbow locked, reverse direction and begin to withdraw it, all the while staying aware of the rest of your body (an important tai chi skill) by maintaining tension.

At the moment that your retracted fist comes to rest, suddenly and completely release all the tension everywhere. This instantaneous transition between maximally tense and maximally relaxed is the most important part of the exploration. In the same way that you paid attention to every muscle in your body when you tensed up, now pay attention to releasing everywhere. Continue letting go until you are on the verge of collapse, maintaining just enough muscle tone to remain in the posture. Now do the same thing on the other side.

Using both hands to repeat the exploration eight times (four times on each side), try to improve body control with each repetition, always paying primary attention to the sudden change from tense to relaxed. Being able to release tension at will is a skill you can use when you are stressed or surprised, such as when a driver suddenly pulls out in front of us, when you receive unexpected bad news, when you find yourself in a conflict—or any other time you feel tight, angry, uncomfortable, or afraid. The more you use it, the more aware you will be of your state of body. Letting go, all the benefits of relaxation come to you.

Bamboo Rings Descend

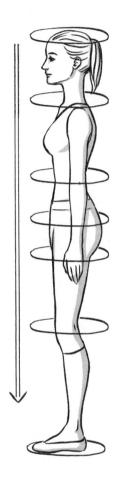

BASED ON TAI CHI'S MEDICAL UNDERPINNINGS AND ADDING an energetic dimension to the muscular work of the previous exercise, this exploration narrows your focus from your whole body to specific sections. As before, begin with your feet shoulder-width apart and fix your attention on the center of the top of your head. Imagine a string starting there, which is the point acupuncturists know as Bai Hui.

Look for a light, floating feeling, then use creative visualization to imagine that your body is segmented from top to bottom by transverse rings as if it were a stalk of bamboo.

Each ring represents a section of the body for you to relax. Start by softening the muscles of your face and neck until your features go slack. Next, focus on the pair of acupuncture points called Jian Jing (Shoulder Well), located in the depressions of the shoulder behind the collarbone. After letting go of any tension there, attend to the paired acupuncture points Zhong Fu (Middle Mansion), which sit in the soft area inside the shoulders and at the very top of the chest. Letting the tension leave this area, breathe deeply, relaxing with your exhaling breath.

Next, move down to the level of the paired Qi Men (Cycle Gate) points a few inches below and in direct line with the nipples. Try to let go of the tension in your upper chest and ribcage. After that, turn your attention to the paired points Zhang Men (Bright Door), which are just to the front of, and below, the bottom rib on each side. This is a critical point for clarity of thinking and for blood pressure as well. Feel the relaxation deeply before proceeding to the next section, defined by the pair of points on the edge of your forearms, in the soft, sensitive depression just in from the elbow and defined by the paired points Qu Qi (Curved Pond). Thinking about softening downward, let your arms drop and relax.

Now attend the point Qi Hai (Sea Qi), which is two finger widths below your navel. Imagine a cross section through this point and the corresponding point at the center of the small of your back, Ming Men (Life Gate). Try to deeply soften the whole body at this lower abdominal level before proceeding to the paired points Qi Chong (Surging Qi). These points are in the front of your body at the inguinal crease. Following this, turn your attention to softening the single point Hui Yin (Merging Perineum) in the middle of the perineum. The sensation is akin to relaxing as if you are preparing to go to the bathroom, but at the same time pulling gently up and in. This a bit of a balancing act, but with practice it will come to you.

Next, relax across the plane defined by the paired Wei Zhong (Popliteal Center) points at the center of the backside of your knees. Be careful not to let your knees buckle as you relax all the way down to the pair of points, Yong Quan (Bubbling Spring), in the middle of the ball of each foot. By the time you reach the bottom, by sequentially relaxing in the fashion of a shaft of bamboo, you have succeeded not only in systematically and deliberately releasing tension you have held for years, but also in dropping your center of gravity and improving your balance. Feel free to repeat this whole sequence as many times as you like.

Shaking

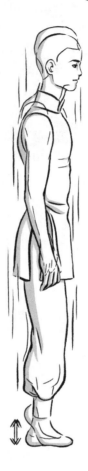

THIS EXPLORATION HAS A BIT TO DO WITH THE LYMPHATIC system, which performs a variety of functions including bolstering the immune system, nourishing tissues, and filtering foreign substances that enter the body from the outside. Filters sometimes need cleaning, and the shaking technique offered here helps. Shaking also helps to reduce tension in the body because, as discussed earlier in the chapter, muscles work in antagonistic pairs—contracting one causes the antagonist to loosen and stretch. Shaking, our muscles get a bit confused and are fooled into cooperating with each other in a special way, thereby reducing tension and increasing flexibility.

Loose and relaxed from the previous explorations, press your teeth gently together so they don't clank against one another or catch your tongue. Now use the muscles in your calves to lift yourself onto your toes and begin with a low frequency, slow bounce. Using your inner awareness to search for any tension that may have crept back in, relax your neck and shoulders, and allow the belly to soften, drawing lightly upward on the perineum as in the previous exploration.

Find a comfortable rhythm and then experiment with gradually increasing the frequency of your shaking, never moving so fast that you become uncomfortable. The first couple of times you shake you may feel the effect of the vibration on your organs. Stop if you become nauseated or dizzy. Over the course of a few weeks of daily practice, build up to five minutes of shaking or more, noticing how it relaxes you and helps chronic muscular tension to fade. In combination with the previous two explorations, this one will produce significant results over time.

Taming the Hot-Rod Heart

Many people find it very stressful to try to keep up with the ongoing deluge of information from the environment and media. The famous psychology researcher and writer, Robert Ornstein, did a study decades ago in which he established that the human brain marks the passage of time on the basis of how much information it receives. A commuter who sees the same scenery rush by the train window every morning finds the ride to work of far lesser duration than his seatmate, who has never taken the ride before. This is because the new rider is fascinated by what he sees, and, paying careful attention, processes more data—the houses, the cars, the people, the river, the rhythm of the wheels, the smell of the vinyl, the click clack of the conductor's ticket punch—than the habitual rider. A rich experience is wonderful, but when the data coming in exceeds our ability to process it we go into an unhealthy overload.

In such an overload—from TV, the Internet, our personal electronic devices—we may even feel we are losing the distinction between what is inside of us and what has not been grasped, between what we actually believe and what we are told, between what we actually experience and what we have seen or heard. This sensory confusion is further complicated by the evolving debate over the nature of the world we think we know. Might reality actually be energy burping into matter, as quantum physicists purport? Is it all an illusion, per many Buddhists? Is it a carefully crafted deception, as portrayed in the movie *The Matrix*? Is it a giant super-organism, as alleged by Deep Ecologists? Is it the all-pervasive thing called nature, as described by the Taoists?

Whatever model we subscribe to, and whether we float around daily on carpets sewn from enlightened thread, push our way onto a subway at rush hour, shower in a tropical rain cloud, or sweat in a coal mine, tai chi can help us to take control of the part of the world we call our own. It can help us find the inner peace and quiet we so desperately crave, even when we do not recognize that burning need for what it is. The very act of participating in something as deliberate, attentive, methodical, introspective, and nurturing as tai chi is quintessentially valuable in our frenetic world. What other activity helps us give our muscles, bones, organs, and joints the attention they deserve? During what other pursuit do we so clearly sense the flow of our thoughts or perceive our role in the tapestry of energy within us and without? When we make it our practice, tai chi can tame our hot-rod hearts and in doing so make the experience of life both deeper and longer.

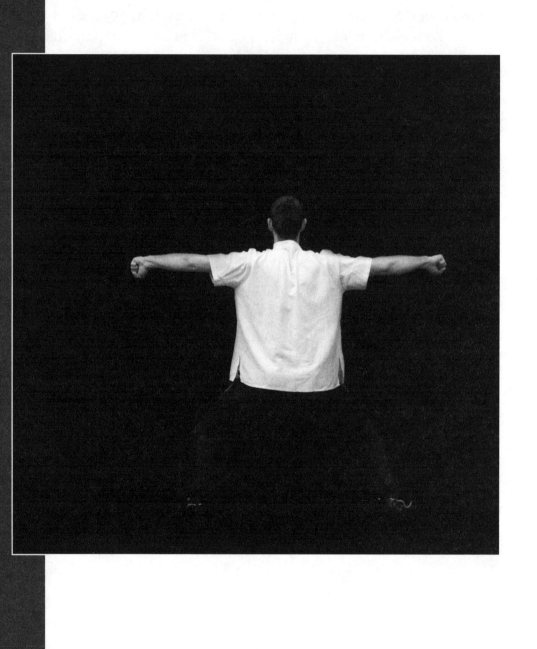

creatures without number
all return to their roots
return to their roots to be still
to be still to revive
to revive to endure
knowing how to endure is wisdom

TAO TE CHING, V.16 (RED PINE, TRANSLATOR)

THE GROUND
BENEATH OUR FEET

In tai chi, connecting with the ground requires rooting, a specific skill that builds upon relaxation and gives us a stable platform from which we can both issue and redirect force. It makes all the sense in the world that tai chi should emphasize our physical connection to the earth, as all Taoist practices have stressed the interconnectedness of all living things on the planet for millennia. In this way, the ancient Taoist originators of tai chi were far ahead of Western thinkers. Our "Green" movement did not start until the 1970s, when Norwegian philosopher Arne Naess coined the phrase "Deep Ecology" to express our connection to the planet that sustains us. Like plants, we grow in a certain soil, are sustained by certain nutrients, and share our space with others whose roots intertwine with our own. Thinking about the culture in which we are raised, the land on which we live, and the people with whom we interact gives us a better understanding of our roots. Tai chi's Chinese forefathers were deeply connected to their land, history, culture, and populace. This chapter explores that connection in terms of our health and our tai chi practice.

THE IMPORTANCE OF ROOTS

Although I had a brick-and-mortar martial arts school in California and have taught at many different indoor venues from hospitals and sports clubs to resorts and even a police department, these days I prefer to indulge tai chi's connection to nature and teach outdoors. My practice is almost always meditative and peaceful, but recently, I found myself martially rooting against a surprise attack in the very Florida park where I conduct many of my classes. It's a lovely place on the water, and although recent hurricanes have stripped it of shade trees and thus concentrated human activity to a few small spots, it is usually a peaceful place.

That particular day, my primary tai chi master arrived from China for a Christmas visit and met me in the park. As he talked and I warmed up, a homeless man approached and asked what I was doing.

"Chinese exercises," I said.

"No you're not. You're doing martial arts. And you know what? I'm going to kick your ass right now."

"Please don't do that."

"I was in the Special Forces," he slurred. "I could just kill you with my bare hands."

My teacher looked uncomfortable, but before the situation could worsen the man shambled away. Drinking tea, we kept easy eyes on him as he made a wide circuit of the park. Absorbed in conversation with my teacher, I stretched in preparation for the day's practice and was just coming out of a deep split when he suddenly changed course and ran at me to throw a punch at the back of my ear.

I will never be sure whether it was the smell of him, the sound of his feet on the grass, or the flicker of surprise on my teacher's face that tipped me off. Whatever the warning, I managed to raise a hand at the very last moment and deflect his attack just before it landed. He sailed past me in a high arc and came to rest some thirty feet away on the concrete seawall.

I rushed to him and found him unconscious, with a bit of blood on his head. Afraid I had killed him, I yelled and slapped his face. His eyelids fluttered and he looked up at me blearily. "What happened?"

"You've been drinking and you fell."

Later, my teacher told me that the reason he had flown so far was that I had been well rooted and met his moment with a spiral touch (more on spiraling in the next chapter) that redirected his force without absorbing any of it. The surprise attack could certainly have gone poorly for me and I was no doubt lucky in my response. As a grace point to the story, I encountered the same homeless man again about two weeks later. Once again he approached and declared his intention to pound me into the ground; this time I answered his challenge differently.

"You tried that once," I said.

He blinked at me. "I did?"

"You punched me in the head. It didn't go well for you."

"I'm sorry."

Weeks later, when I saw him again, he sat down and told me a great deal about his military experience, the people he had killed, his alienation from his family, and how things had fallen apart for him. Closer, I saw that he was riddled with disease, and that despite my offers to help, he was not long for this world. I never saw him again.

PALM TREES, GRAVITY, EARTH, AND SPACE

The story brings into sharp focus at least two distinct aspects of rooting. The first is the importance of the nurturing roots of friends and family that had obviously failed my attacker. The second relevant aspect of the story is my attacker's insensitivity to the earth energies at work upon him, especially the ubiquitous force of gravity. Without gravity we would have nothing to push against, nothing to give us a direction into which to drop our iron lollipop, nothing to provide a link between relaxation and rooting. Gravity allowed me to create an energy conduit between the ground and his fist so that my tai chi deflection was effective.

Relaxation, through gravity, necessarily leads to rooting. Relaxing, we drop our center of gravity. Dropping our center of gravity, we can actually feel the pressure on our feet as we meld with the ground. Indeed quantum physics tells us that the hard surfaces of matter we appreciate are a matter of probability only, that if all variables cooperated our hand could go through a wall without impact and our feet could sink all the way to the earth's core without a scratch. Perhaps that's why we feel stickiness between our feet and the ground when we root. Of course rooting relies on Newtonian physics, too. Tai chi works because the ground offers us an equal and opposite reaction to the forces acting upon us. That's why the art doesn't work so well in space; absent gravity, we have nothing to push against.

Rooting, we relate to the world as a tree does, albeit a very mobile one. Our feet and their connection to the ground are the roots, our hips and legs are the trunk, and our torso is the crown of the tree, dancing in the wind, light and responsive, ready to willingly, even joyfully bend to incoming force. Like the tree, we must foster our roots, strengthen our trunk, and yet find in our sinking and our relaxation the ability to sway with the wind, to anticipate and neutralize pushes, grabs, locks, shoves, kicks, and punches by yielding, though not by giving up. A tree that gives up snaps and breaks. A person who cannot stay soft, relaxed, and loose—who cannot manage the unique tai chi blend of strength lower down and lightness and grace above—will be overcome. Like dancing branches we must turn, twist, writhe, spiral and bend, all the while maintaining our sense of self and our place in the world. As tai chi players, we are able to handle the proverbial slings and arrows of outrageous fortune by acting like trees.

The tree is such a successful biological formula that nature has provided us with so many arboreal examples of well-rooted trees perfectly adapted to their specific environments. The giant African Baobab survives droughts and desert windstorms with strong roots and a small crown, the mighty Sequoia intertwines with other trees to root both above and below in coastal gales, the familiar palm bends nearly horizontal in hurricanes but roots so well it stays planted. In a sense, all trees are natural tai chi players.

All phases of tai chi practice—forms, solo exercises (single moves repeated), partner exercises, and meditation—require us to root just as they require us to embody the art's other important principles. In every movement we consciously relax, sink, and grab the ground with our heels and toes. Our upper body yields to incoming force while we activate our hips in the very specific way described in a later chapter. Over time and with consistent effort we discover for ourselves that rooting is a blend of ideation, emotional state, and physical prowess. We must learn how to use it, groom it, and grow it until it is an asset as steady and companionable as our skin.

THE LESS TANGIBLE ROOTS OF TAI CHI LINEAGE AND TRADITION

Our modern practice is inspired by the traditional Chinese cultural celebration of ancestors and the work they have done to get us where we are. In tai chi terms, this means we pay homage to lineage, myths, legends, training manuals, and philosophical treatises. While in the West we are more likely to speak of influences and schools than of disciples and character, in kung fu culture the term lineage implies keeping secrets from outsiders while sharing them with disciples, so-called "indoor" students, often family. This tradition not only preserves the art but makes sure that life-and-death information is purposefully given only into the right hands. Whether you are learning tai chi from a famous master, in a kung fu school, in a community center, or even from a part-time instructor in a park, you are being taught an organic practice that has grown up from the soil of twenty generations of a particular Chinese family, and before that scores of dynasties worth of scholarship and experience.

My own primary teacher, Master Max Yan, is proud of the recent roots that connect him to tai chi's founding Chen family of Chenjiagou, Henan Province, China, and the older ones that link him directly to the rulers of the State of Yan, a northeastern kingdom that was one of the more important city–states of the Eastern Zhou Dynasty's so-called Warring States period. In addition to possessing physical genius, Master Yan is a man of extraordinary intellect and a deep sense of history and tradition. Each and every tai chi concept he has transmitted to me drips with authentic Chinese culture and hundreds of years of Chen family nuance and expertise. Without it, my understanding would be paltry.

Any legitimate teacher will be eager to share details of her lineage, and often to share stories, too. I know many anecdotes about Master Yan. One of my favorites is that after proving, at 125 lbs, that giant professional football players could not budge him one inch, he was hired as an assistant coach by the Miami Dolphins football team and given the task of teaching defensive players the same skill. Apparently even the NFL understands the value of rooting.

Rooting exercises require introspection and quiet sensitivity. Helping you to pay attention to your body in new and specific ways, they are good training for other challenging explorations offered later in this book. Stay focused, and treat these explorations like a joy-filled puzzle that allows you to test the limits of what you are able to accomplish when mind and body work together.

Transmitting Force to the Ground

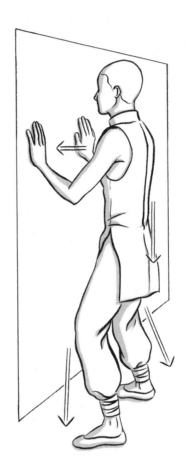

FACING A WALL, RELAX YOUR SHOULDERS AND LET YOUR ARMS hang down. Positioning your feet at shoulder width, grip the ground with your toes and dig in your heels. Imagine a string from heaven lifting your head and straightening your back as you sink into your hips and fill your lumbar spine until it is flat. Gently exhale as you hollow your chest and drop your breastbone down and back in the direction of your tailbone. Place your hands on the wall, adjusting your stance if you need to so that your elbows remain pointed down and unlocked.

Without leaning into it, begin pushing on the wall. Keep your spine vertical and distribute your weight evenly across your feet, neither rocking back onto your heels nor shifting forward into your toes. Sinking into the ground and continuing to push, release all tension from your chest. If you find it difficult to relax while pushing, ease up on the force a bit and then try again. The idea is to borrow power from the ground rather than from your muscles, and to feel the bidirectional nature of the force. In a sense, you push on the wall and the wall pushes back on you.

Try changing your body position to see how the force changes with it. If you turn your toes inward can you still conduct force to the floor effectively and without discomfort? What about if you turn them outward, lock your hips, arch your pelvis, bend back excessively, or lift one or both shoulders? In each case these violations of correct alignment affect your ability to connect with the ground. The more familiar you become with what it takes to align yourself properly when receiving or issuing force, the better your rooting will be.

In addition to good alignment, rooting requires a calm, clear mind. Negative emotions such as anger, sadness, frustration, distraction, or agitation affect your body's ability to effortlessly transmit force. Test this assertion by thinking of something that makes you angry while doing the exercise. Do you notice the resultant prickle of perspiration in your palms and overall rise in your tension? Can you feel how you have to work harder when pushing at the wall in this state? Try thinking of something that makes you sad. Do you notice how the wall suddenly seems stronger? Play with other emotions. Doing so will improve your understanding of how rooting well helps you to manage force. See if you can bring your new awareness into play in your everyday life, doing your best to keep combative and stressful thoughts away so as to remain powerfully rooted in your world.

Rooting Through Angles

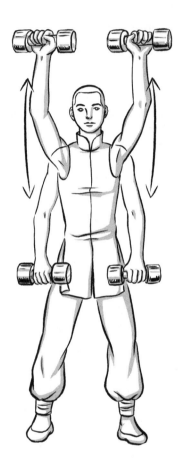

THIS EXERCISE USES A DUMBBELL AS A SUBSTITUTE FOR A WALL
so that you can learn about the relationship between body alignment
and the angle at which force (in this case, weight) is applied. If you're
new to exercise, start with a weight of 2 lbs. If you're a seasoned athlete or bodybuilder, use a heavier weight of up to 20 lbs.

Start with your feet shoulder-width apart. Hold the dumbbell in front of you with your arms straight and elbows not quite locked. Now lift it slowly up over your head. As you do, concentrate on feeling all the different muscle groups involved. Try to stay relaxed and connected to the ground. If you feel a burn in your shoulders, see if you can relax to release it, allowing the force the dumbbell and gravity generate together to go straight through your body and into the ground. Notice the changes in the pressure on your feet. Can you feel force more in your heels or more in your toes? Adjust so that the entire foot contacts the ground evenly. As you slowly lower the weight, pay attention to the way your body compensates for the new directions of the force. Don't lean at all. Keep your spine straight.

Next, try slowly lifting the dumbbell out to the side, using one hand. Go as high as you can without hurting your shoulder, changing the angles to explore how your body reacts. Maintain good alignment and relaxed muscles as you do. Once you get the hang of moving the weight around while keeping an even contact patch between your feet and the ground, you can experiment with moving the weight more quickly. Over the course of a week or two of daily practice, you should be able to adapt readily to different angles and different speeds.

Remember to keep the small of your back flat and your chest and shoulders relaxed. Feel your hips move subtly in response to the shifting weight. In tai chi we learn to disconnect our emotions from the force being applied to us, and to calmly adjust our level of tension and the angles of our structure to accommodate and redirect the force with maximal efficiency and minimum effort. As the weight rises and falls we should function like a pipe carrying water, relying on our structure to do the work as opposed to our muscles.

Rooting with a Partner

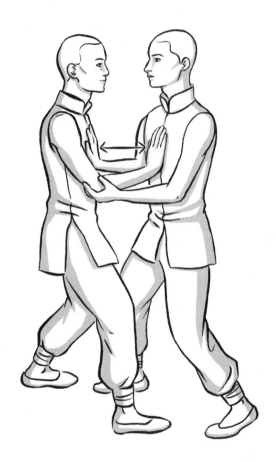

NOW THAT YOU HAVE TRIED PUSHING AGAINST AN INANIMATE object and moving weight, the next step is to work with another person. Ideally, you want to work with someone of approximately your own height and weight. More, because partner work can try your patience and challenge your ego, you also want someone who is patient, centered, and eager to learn rather than show off. Conflict in what should be a cooperative environment will slow your progress, so choosing the right partner is essential.

Face your partner with your right foot forward and your left foot behind. Adjust your alignment to each other so that your right foot is beside your partner's. Place your right palm with its fingertips upward on your partner's breastbone, and have him do the same for you. Your left hand cups your partner's right elbow from beneath, while your partner's left hand cups your left elbow in the same fashion. In this mutually agreeable position, ask your partner to begin to apply pressure to your breastbone. The greater the pressure, the more you must relax and root, noticing the qualitative difference between a force you initiate yourself and one that comes from someone else. Relax, check your shoulders, maintain a straight spine, and keep your hips loose. Ask your partner to angle her push slightly upward. This additional challenge will require you to relax and root even more.

Once you get the hang of handling a straight push, ask your partner to make things more challenging by turning her hand to make the push more challenging. After that, you may want to move the position of the hand to the belly or the hip. The lower the push, the more difficult it can be to relax into it and not lose your balance, as low pushes are closer to our center of gravity. You can ask your partner to make things even more difficult for you by simultaneously pushing with one hand and using her grip on your elbow to pull you backward or sideways. All these pushes and pulls should be slow and gentle at first so that your body can understand the game. If you both agree, you can step things up a bit and see how you do. Use your hands like sensory instruments, not only returning your partner's force when she agrees to receive it, but also detecting her intention at the earliest possible moment. The sooner you know what force is coming, the better equipped to deal with it you will be.

As a final wrinkle, experiment with emotions as you did in the solo exercise. Tell your partner a joke and then give a push while she is laughing. Have your partner tell you a sad story and see what happens to your ability to handle force when your concentration is interrupted. See if you can use this cooperative exploration of rooting to discover all those variables that contribute to you being able to take force to the ground without losing your balance, to be able to root like a tree even in a strong and changeable wind.

Rooted in a Wondrous Past

All three legs of the tripod upon which tai chi rests—medicine, philosophy, and indigenous martial arts—penetrate deep into China's history and soil, and are historically linked to each other in a way that bolsters tai chi's foundation. Much of the first leg, what Westerners now call Traditional Chinese Medicine, was lost during Mao Zedong's so-called Cultural Revolution. What remains is actually a ghost of a much larger, deeper, and more intricate body of knowledge that existed at least a thousand years before the nation we now know as China came into being.

The second leg, Taoist philosophy harkens back to the beginning of the Xia Dynasty (2194 B.C.E.) and China's Bronze Age, when shamans used Taoist methods to predict the future by charting the course of rivers, following the paths of clouds, smelling the wind, and learning the habits of fish, birds, and bees. While ancient by the standards of most world cultures, even tai chi's philosophical handbook, Lao Tzu's *Tao Te Ching*, is a relatively recent work in the context of Taoism's long history. Penned by one or more authors about 500 B.C.E., some consider it a commentary on the much older Yiqing (I-*Ching*, *Book of Changes*), written some 600 years earlier.

Indigenous martial arts comprise the third leg of the tai chi tripod. Academically called neigong, they can be traced back to mythical figures of China's prehistory such as the famed Yellow Emperor. The thirteenth century figure Zhang Sanfeng is reputed to be the father of arts leading to the one recently named tai chi ch'uan. Those wishing to suggest tai chi's origins are elsewhere may challenge the existence of this Song Dynasty internal martial arts sage, though there is real evidence that Zhang (Chinese put surnames first, given names second) existed, as he left behind written works. Although few of these have been translated into English, a Qing-Dynasty scholar named Li Xiyue collected some of them into a book entitled the *Complete Works of Gentleman Zhang Sanfeng*, which is, in turn, preserved in the *Selections of the Taoist Canon*.

Zhang is thought to have developed his system on China's famed Wudang Mountain, a mecca to modern martial artists and one of Taoism's most important sites. Wudang's geologic and geographic qualities evoke the archetypal mountain scenes so often rendered in classical Chinese paintings. The Wudang mountain complex, which spans nearly 150 square miles and includes lakes, rivers, waterfalls, 72 peaks, as many rock temples, and a forest that to this day sustains more than 600 Chinese herbs. Given the importance of water in Taoist thought and tai chi practice alike, Wudang makes perfect sense as the inspirational home of tai chi.

The practice of neigong on Wudang is well documented and stretches back millennia. In fact, "wu" means martial and "dang" means resistance. Unsurprisingly, Wudang has a tremendous military history. As long ago as the Zhou Dynasty's Spring and Autumn Period (between the eighth and fourth centuries B.C.E.), the mountain was located in the state of Chu, whose armies relied on their martial skills to successfully fend off the attacks of neighboring Qin, the all-conquering kingdom that would eventually unify China.

We may not be able to say that Chu's soldiers used tai chi but we can say that the art arose in recognizable form in the early 1600s through a collaboration, at a place called Qianzai Temple, between the sixteenth-century general Chen Wang Ting and two brothers, Li Zhong and Li Xin, after the Chen and Li families intermarried. Perhaps coincidentally, Li is the surname of Lao Tzu, presumed author of the *Tao Te Ching*. The Chen-Li brothers' system was refined some thirty miles from Qianzai in Henan province at the Chen family village, known as Chenjiaguo. Since the early 1600s, tai chi has been preserved, deepened, and refined there. While the Chen family version is the original, traditional version of the art we now call tai chi, derivative versions have become popular. Among others, these include the widely practiced Yang style, two styles that go by the name of Wu, and Sun style, which is a combination of tai chi and another internal martial art, Baguazhang.

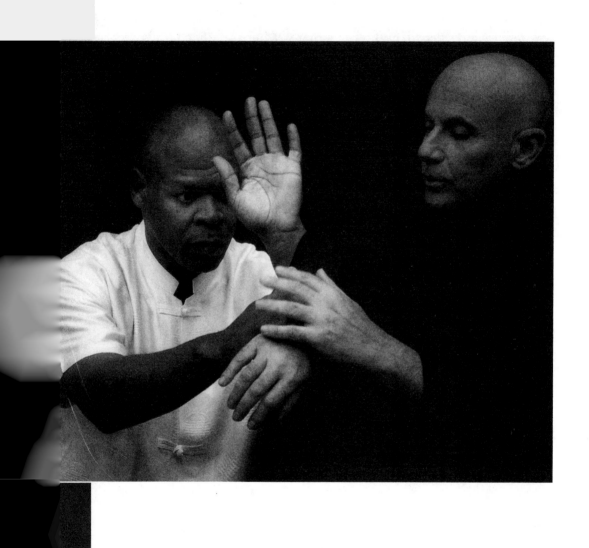

3

When life begins
We are tender and weak
When life ends
We are still and rigid
All things, including the grass and trees,
Are soft and pliable in life
Dry and brittle in death

TAO TE CHING, V.76 (JONATHAN STARR, TRANSLATOR)

SECRETS, SPIRALS, MINDFULNESS, AND WATER

There are various reasons why tai chi exercise changes the body in unique ways and develops unique skills. Among these is the fact that the movements themselves have a certain unique character. Reflecting its Taoist founder's passion for watching and learning from nature, tai chi players spiral like whirlpools and flow like water. This chapter will offer a clearer picture of what those oft-cited terms really mean. We will explore what tai chi movements look and feel like, as well as their intended martial purpose. Even if we have no interest in tai chi for physical self-defense, knowing the purpose of a movement is invaluable in performing it correctly.

Before we have any experience with the art, many of us move as if made of two big glass marbles, one sitting atop the other in a jar full of glue. During the first year of practice the glue turns to honey and the marbles shrink and multiply as we learn to sink, relax, and turn. After another year or two of practice the honey becomes less viscous and our marbles become polished ball bearings, making every gesture more subtle and our foundation stable. Little by little, and with more time and practice, we reduce our ball bearings to sand. Newly dense and precise in our movements, we quiet our mind with meditation until we can feel how the turning of even one grain of sand affects the rest.

At the master level, the quantitative changes we have enjoyed become qualitative. Rather than working with a body made of solid bits, we move as if we are pure water. Thus transformed we experience the miracles so many long-term players report: the disappearance of life-long aches and pains, the easing or even cure of long-term chronic conditions, the minimizing of negative emotions, the increase in concentration, the sharpening of focus, and the rise of non-dual perception as the illusion of separation from the world around us fades.

A SPECIAL TWIST ON FLEXIBILITY

Despite the metaphorical phase change between solid and liquid, one dynamic of tai chi movement remains constant as we advance: the tai chi player must follow that most archetypal of all nature's three-dimensional designs, the spiral. There are many other ways in which tai chi owes a debt to nature, but there is no clearer example of the art's natural underpinnings than that marvelous shape, which is seen in galaxies, the chambered nautilus, and in hurricanes, tornadoes, and waterspouts. The spiral is truly the quintessential shape of tai chi.

Perhaps you remember the balsawood toy airplane from long ago. Packaged flat and originally selling for less than a dollar, it featured a plastic propeller, wooden wings, and derived the power for flight from a rubber band. Upon first assembly, the rubber band needed to be stretched between the propeller and a metal hook at the tail, but after repeated use, the rubber band was far more relaxed. This stretching of the rubber band happened because winding the band made first one row of knots in the band, then another upon that row, and then—if you were willing to risk breaking the band in search of greater performance—a third upon that.

What does a balsa toy teach us about tai chi? Well, a twist is just another word for a spiral and when we spiral the band we also stretch it. Rather than linear stretching, as is commonly done in sports warm-ups and many forms of yoga, tai chi exerts a spiraling force on connective tissue, stabilizer muscles, and major muscle groups. Stretching our tissues to their straight-line limits, we run the risk of tears. Twisting them, however, we are more likely to feel those limits because the process is more gradual and there is more time for feedback from the tissues. More, the twisting movement itself is easier on muscle fibers, as smaller bundles are engaged serially rather than the whole muscle at one time. Stretching with nature's spiral, it turns out, is just as effective as the straight line pull, and safer, too.

THE TOWEL, THE CORKSCREW, AND THE SPINE

Other than tossing it into the clothes dryer, the best way to get the water out of a wet towel is not to slap or stomp on it, but to wring it with a twisting motion. In general, moving liquid through a solid medium is well accomplished with spirals, a fact known in the field of fluid dynamics. One of the reasons that tai chi movements prove beneficial to organs, muscles, and joints is that spirals push blood through tissue just the way we wring water from a towel.

In order to better understand the requirements of tai chi spiraling, we might draw a parallel between the human body and the corkscrew, which also requires a particular combination of precise alignment and correct motion in order to operate successfully. The first requirement in using a corkscrew correctly is that it be applied vertically. If we position it at an angle, it will end up against the inside of the neck of the bottle rather than in the cork. Pulling up on it will merely destroy the cork if it has not bitten centered and true. In addition, when we use a corkscrew we must turn it. If we don't, we will force the cork down into the wine. Last, we must apply downward pressure, for if we simply turn a straight corkscrew we will do no more than create a divot on the surface of the cork.

As for the corkscrew, so for the tai chi player. Our spine must remain straight, we must sink and relax, and we must turn. Turning occurs at the waist and in the hips, but not in the knees, which are designed to bend but not twist. Imagining a long drill bit attached to the tailbone and spiraling down into the ground and you have the picture of the spine acting as the axis of the drill. Of course our tai chi body is not a single corkscrew, but many. Each limb is a corkscrew, and each digit a corkscrew, too, allowing for a great number of different-sized spirals simultaneously acting in different planes and directions. As we proceed along the previously described continuum from giant marbles to water, the spirals in our body become more complex, numerous, and subtle.

THE GYROSCOPE WE CALL DANTIAN

To spiral as powerfully as water, which overcomes snags and obstructions by simply flowing around them in three-dimensional fashion, we must train our muscular core to turn like that perennial favorite toy, the spinning gyroscope. Typically, the toy gyroscope is comprised of a metal cage inside of which a rotor spins on an axle. There is a hole in the axle for a piece of string. We wind the string around the axle, give a good pull to spin the rotor, and then set the cage down on its end. The inertia of the spinning rotor allows the toy to balance on its tip. If we pick up the top and turn it in our hands, we can feel the way it resists our efforts to move it in any axis other than the axis of the spin.

This resistance is a quality that has made the gyroscope of great commercial importance. Airplanes use gyros in their instruments and ships ranging in size from private yachts to supertankers use gyros—

called stabilizers—to counter the effects of rough seas. The latter are positioned at various angles and linked to sensors and computer controlled so as to present a complex, effective response to the pitch and yaw of a ship, as well as the roll. Driven by electric motors, ship gyros speed up in rough seas and slow down when it is calm, thereby matching the forces acting upon them.

During tai chi practice, our pelvic girdle and hip joints—and the muscles that drive them—create a functional unit that acts like a natural gyro, turning at different speeds at different angles and with different force according as needed. The Chinese call this combination of energy, joint, meat, and bone the Dantian, and consider it the power center of the body, and the center of mass, too. Our biggest muscle groups, the hamstrings and quads, support the area. Spiraling, turning, and sinking, the properly rotating tai chi Dantian does for us in the storm of life just what a ship's stabilizers do in a challenging sea.

Tai chi training strengthens and refines this magnificent asset for use not only in martial practice but in other areas of life as well. Any and every activity of our daily routine can be made easier by proper use of our Dantian, including mowing the lawn, doing laundry, opening a cabinet, cooking, bicycling, carrying a child, taking out the trash, planting a garden, and even driving a car. All that is needed is the right training and the right mental connections and we can create stability for ourselves as well as accomplish great physical work.

WATERING YOUR MIND

Discipline, devotion to the art, hard work, and much practice should be enough to transform our mind/body in tai chi fashion, but they are not. There are millions of people in China and other Asian nations who rise every morning and do their form in the park simply out of habit. It's part of their daily routine, part of their culture, part of their lives, and yet they are still not gaining nearly as much benefit as they could. Similarly, there are people in this country who practice their forms every day for years, people who may even learn to masterfully wield a tai chi spear or lunge impressively with a tai chi straight sword, but who never achieve the inner connection that really makes the art function at its highest level. How can this be?

The answer is that there are two ways to play tai chi. We can treat the art as a regular workout—like calisthenics, say, or a set of tennis—and go through the motions as best we can, building our buns and thighs with low stances while treating the sequence of moves, the form, as just one more way to move the body, perhaps in a social setting. Alternately, we can perform the practice mindfully, paying attention to every move and going deep inside ourselves. Fending off the speed-and-greed messages of the media-driven world around us, we practice until the universe contracts to a single, focused doorway to a reality greater than we can possibly imagine. Mindful practice increases our sensitivity, calm, awareness of our surroundings, and understanding of the true nature of our body, which is, variously, an assemblage of co-operating microorganisms, a series of independent linked systems, or a unified whole born of millions of years of evolution and expressing a complex consciousness.

Researchers are discovering that one of the ways in which our brains are capable of storing and accessing so much information—of melding memories and making creative leaps and associations—is by forming branching connections where neurons meet. Such electro-chemical connections—the results of our experience, particularly when multiple senses are involved—actually create physical changes in our brain. The more "global" our learning (meaning the more we physically experience the lesson rather than just hearing about it) the more lasting and transformative that lesson invariably is.

Mindful tai chi practice thus builds awareness and sensitivity to our environment and helps us to notice where we have difficulties dealing with force (not enough spiraling), lose our balance easily (not enough root), or feel tension and fatigue (not enough relaxation). This last is especially important in tai chi, for all that is powerful and good in the art requires strong softness. Places we commonly hold tension include the neck, the low back, the jaw, the shoulders, and the hips. Many men also hold tension in a flat, pyramid-shaped chunk of muscle embedded deep in our gluteal region. This piriform muscle, which functions to open the hip joint laterally, is rarely used in our sedentary lifestyle and is tough to stretch because of its position among other large muscles in the rear end.

Over time, particularly in men of middle years, the piriform muscle may become foreshortened and tight, reducing the mobility of the hip joint and sometimes even contributing to the radiating pain known as sciatica. Since tai chi uses spiral motion to stretch the muscles in question, the internal focus of the practice can make us aware of this muscle, which many of us never even knew existed. Becoming aware of it, we lessen chronic pain by stretching and relaxing it. We also gain increased range of motion in the hips, which empowers our tai chi movements by improving the function of the Dantian.

There are many other examples of an aware mind leading to physical change. If we train our mind to notice particular problems without getting stuck on them, we can generate power like water, which, while yielding to the touch, can also cut rock, capsize oil tankers, and flood coastal cities. Moving with the grace and fluidity of water means using our stronger bits to support our weaker bits until they, too, can strengthen, while all the while protecting them from injury.

TOP-SECRET TAI CHI MOVEMENTS AND ENERGIES

Martial tai chi (technically, tai chi ch'uan) was conceived in the days before satellites and cruise missiles. Knowing how to fight was a key to survival in those early days, and a key to livelihood too. The Chen family, developers of the art we practice today, were highly regarded as bodyguards by both rulers and wealthy merchants. In addition to offering personal protection against assassins, Chen tai chi masters provided protection for caravans of goods traveling down bandit-infested roads.

Over time, it became clear that those who practiced tai chi were not only skilled soldiers and fighters but lived long and healthy lives. As tai chi's health benefits became increasingly manifest, the Chen family guarded the art's special knowledge and skills ever more closely, transmitting the information only to family members and most trusted disciples. During the years after Mao Zedong's "Cultural Revolution," all that changed. It was no longer socially acceptable to withhold secrets from others in this flagrant fashion. The holders of tai chi's innermost secrets were faced with a choice—spill the beans or be sent to a "re-education" camps where people were frequently tortured to death.

The art of tai chi is all about finding creative solutions, and during that difficult time in Chinese history, the beleaguered tai chi masters found one. Outwardly, they tailored their practice to match official guidelines; in secret they persisted in practicing and teaching tai chi's politically incorrect fighting core. Seeing themselves as guardians of information that had at one time been critical to the survival of their friends and families—and, they reasoned, might be again some time in the future—they obscured the true art any way they could on the outside while preserving it behind closed doors. It was this, the old masters must have concluded, or lose the art forever.

Spiral movement is one thing they were determined not to lose; yet ironically it is being lost anyway. This is because the martial core of the art, its original purpose, has been replaced by a greater interest in the art's health benefits. While this makes the art a great blessing to a wider range of people than were previously even aware of its existence, it also threatens the integrity of the art. One of the marvelous things about tai chi movements and principles is that we can test them. The test may be friendly and cooperative, but it is still a test. If what we are doing does not work martially, it may be incorrect. If it is incorrect, it will not provide the maximal health benefit.

As popular practice moves farther and farther away from martial application, a tai chi gumbo has arisen. Some of the ingredients in this muddy soup were put into the original stockpot so as to purposely obfuscate closely held fighting techniques. More were added later as a result of misunderstanding the original material. Since spiral movement is one of the most important secrets of the art, a great deal of confusion has arisen over what it is, what it means, how to do it, and how to use it.

Over the years, I have variously seen the two-dimensional components of a spiral (directions of movement that create a three dimensional spiral when combined) called Pluck, Pull, Roll Back, Squeeze, Press, Spit, Float, Sink, Swallow, the "prow of the boat," and more. While some advocates of these terms and interpretations may well have a deep understanding of the practice, such words (like the thirteen so-called intrinsic energies of tai chi—including receiving, neutralizing, enticing, issuing, borrowing, sinking) do little to reveal how to spiral.

Fortunately, there are four short words, each of which describes direction of movement relative to the center of a practitioner's body, that together paint a clear, spiral picture. The first of these words is Peng (pronounced "pung"). To understand Peng, we might imagine holding the axle of a bicycle wheel between the fingers of two hands. The wheel is in a vertical plane (as it would be on the road) and the tire valve is next to our breastbone. To start the Peng movement we spin the wheel so that the tire valve goes down toward the ground and comes up again on the side of the wheel that is away from us. The first-down-and-then-up path of the valve is Peng.

As simple as it sounds, the direction of movement we call Peng has powerful ramifications to our tai chi practice. Because it starts close to you, goes down, and then comes up, Peng lifts the opponent. Deprived of his connection to the ground he has nothing to push off against. This weakens whatever attacks he can manage while trying not to fall down, rendering him virtually harmless. Peng is the most martially important of the four directions of movement precisely because it addresses a practitioner's first and overarching concern—his safety. Please remember, we don't have to care about using tai chi to fight to benefit from these explanations. It's just that considering a movement's original purpose makes it so much clearer.

If, while holding the bicycle wheel in our hands again, we spin it so that the valve—again starting by our breastbone and rotating in a vertical plane—goes up first and then down, we have described An (pronounced "ahn"), the second direction of movement. Where Peng is the bottom half of a vertical circle, An is the top half. Where Peng lifts an opponent and throws him away, An unbalances him, then drives him into the ground. We can use Peng to send a training partner on an enjoyable "flight"; the Internet is full of videos of tai chi players doing exactly this. An, by contrast, is a conversation stopper and no fun at all, as it leaves a partner on the ground at your feet.

Remember, Peng and An take place only in the vertical plane. To create a three-dimensional spiral we must add the horizontal plane to our movements, and for that we turn to the third direction of movement, Ji (pronounced "jee"). To understand Ji, let's ditch our bicycle wheel in favor of another useful and common object—the rotating serving plate called the Lazy Susan. Set in the middle of a dinner table, this device allows us to pass food to one another easily. If the person across the table asks for the broccoli, all we have to do is spin the Lazy Susan and presto, broccoli delivered. Whenever the broccoli is circling away from us (either to the left or the right) in this horizontal plane, we call the direction of its movement Ji.

We have only one direction of movement left to explore, and that is Liu (pronounced "lyoo"). Having already wrapped our mind around the concept of circles and spirals, vertical and horizontal planes, this last one is easy. Liu describes the direction of motion of receiving the broccoli. When we ask someone to pass it to us on the Lazy Susan, whether it comes in from the left or comes in from the right, the direction of movement is Liu.

Each of these elementary directions describes half of a circle, and with its dimensional partner a full circle. Each pair of movements defines a geometric plane. Life, however, does not happen in two dimensions, but in three. We get those dimensions when we tilt the bike wheel to one side or the other, or when we lift one end of the Lazy Susan. Combining the horizontal and the vertical dimensions into myriad combinations, we are mixing up Peng, Liu, Ji, and An.

Those mixtures are spirals, and the tai chi player's ability to execute them improves with time and practice. Like marbles turning to bearings, sand, and eventually water, the spirals that begin as simple movements of the arms come to involve not only our muscular core but also our tendons, ligaments, and bones. More, as our tai chi level improves, the spirals decrease in size while they increase in complexity, leading to better circulation of blood, lymph, and qi, as well as greater martial effectiveness.

Sophisticated spirals require relaxation, practice, and correct instruction. They also require a quiet mind able to develop the body by paying attention to the little cues that come in, and to respond to external forces with awareness, equanimity, and relaxation. Eventually, when the spirals become sufficiently small and subtle, they can no longer be seen. At this point they are said to be energies rather than mere mechanical devices, abiding in the body at rest but ready at any moment to manifest in response to an attacker's force.

Noticing a connection between the way a silkworm produces silk and the spirals we have been discussing, masters of yore gave tai chi spiraling movement the name Chan Si Jin (pronounced "chan su djin") or "Silk Reeling." Today we recognize that silk reeling depends upon varying proportions of Peng, Liu, Ji, and An, and must pervade every movement we make in our practice. Unique to authentic, traditional tai chi, Silk Reeling demands training of both mind and body, and differentiates the art from any other.

Straight Line Vs. Spiral

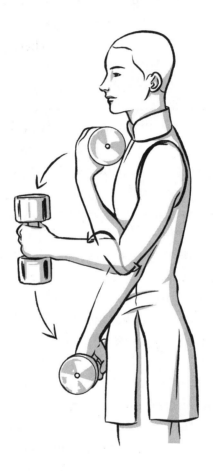

MOVING IN A SPIRAL ENGAGES MUSCLES DIFFERENTLY THAN moving in a straight line. Using a dumbbell can help you feel this difference. The weight should be slightly challenging, but not uncomfortable. As before, choose a weight between 2 and 20 lbs, according to your strength and fitness level. Now stand with your feet shoulder-width apart and execute a straight curl, beginning with the weight at our side, palm forward, then lifting it up to your shoulder while keeping the elbow pointed down. Make sure to avoid turning the wrist. Return the weight to your side in the reverse movement. You could think of the pair of movements, the raising and lowering, as curling and uncurling. When you cannot manage even one more full curl, make note of how many curls you did and where you feel any muscle soreness or joint stiffness. Repeat the exercise using your other arm.

After a suitable rest period (how long depends upon your physical condition and your age, but ten minutes should be enough to allow any soreness to fade), curl the same dumbbell from the same starting position, except that instead of having your palm face forward, turn it around so your palm faces to the rear. The weight should follow the centerline of your body. Keep your elbow pointed down and rotate your forearm along its long axis, spiraling the weight as you lift it until it has turned as far as you can turn it. When you can't do even one more curl, again note the number of curls you did and where you feel any muscle soreness or weakness. After another rest period, try increasing the weight by 25 percent in both exercises. Repeat the exercise on the other side. At some point you will notice that because you are recruiting more muscles, you can lift a heavier weight when you spiral than you can when you do a straight curl.

Spirals in Our Joints

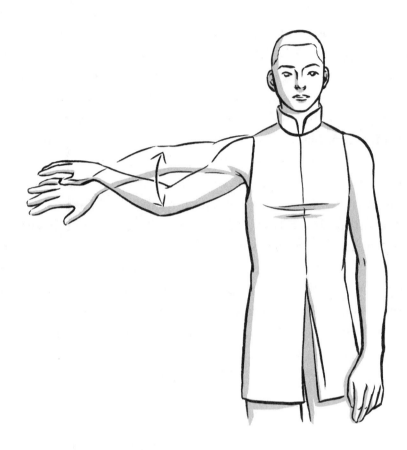

IN THIS EXERCISE YOU WILL EXPERIENCE THE SPECIFIC EFFECT of spiraling on the shoulder, elbow, and wrist. Begin by standing with your feet shoulder-width apart, your arms by your sides, your shoulders down and relaxed, and your spine straight and head erect as if being held by a string from heaven. Now raise your left arm out to our side. Keeping your shoulder down and relaxed, rotate your elbow so that it points at the floor while keeping the palm facing downward. If you feel any sense of strain in your shoulder, check and make sure that your breastbone is dropped and your shoulder blades don't protrude. Once you manage this technique with the left arm, repeat it with the right. Last, perform the movement with both arms simultaneously. This will be easier if you can keep your breastbone sunken inward, your lower back dropped, and your tailbone tucked under.

This may be the first time you've thought about the effect a seemingly isolated movement has on the rest of the body. Cultivating a new awareness of the integration of the body is the purpose of this exercise, as such integration is a critical aspect of physical practice. Using our structure to avoid injury and connect force with the ground is what allows us to contend with opponents bigger than we are. More, allowing force to pass through us is a skill that spares our feelings as well as our muscles and bones, thereby lessening the effects of insults, stress, turns of ill fortune, and the ravages of disease.

Spirals Contending with Force

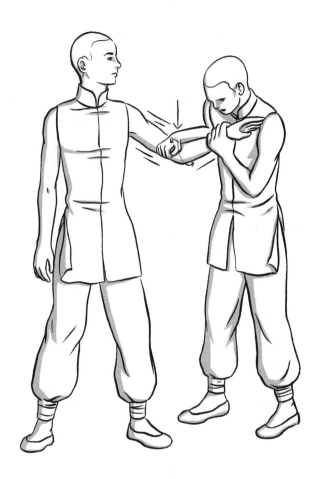

THIS EXPLORATION REQUIRES THE ASSISTANCE OF ONE PARTNER and is even better with two. As before, pick people who are cooperative, have an easy disposition, and are interested in learning about tai chi body dynamics. Once again, begin with your feet shoulder-width apart. Extend your right arm out to the side again, and without performing the spiral ask your partner to take your hand and use your arm to bend your elbow. Even if you resist, your partner is likely able to succeed if he uses both hands. Do the same exercise on the other side.

Now try resisting using the spiral you practiced in the last exploration. Keep your shoulders down and relaxed, soften your chest, drop your lower back, extend your arm so that your palm and elbow are down. In addition to performing the physical spiral, put your mind into it. Imagine the currents of blood spiraling through your arm. Imagine the muscles turning under your skin. Let the spiral connect not only your palm and your shoulder, but your shoulder and your feet, passing like a wave all the way through your body. The difference in your strength should be apparent to both of you.

As a last step in this exploration, ask a second partner to help by working the other arm at the same time. Challenged by forces on both sides, you have to be doubly good at taking force to the ground to contend with this exercise. Notice what happens when you try. Do you feel your attention jumping from one arm to the other? Successfully resisting attacks on both your arms at the same time gives you a taste of the multitude of spirals tai chi training creates. It also cultivates a level of awareness that will eventually extend to the entire body.

Taoist Masters and Tai Chi

Tai chi is based on philosophical Taoism, a way of looking at the world distinct from Taoist religion, a popular, pantheistic, animist movement with many sects that arose sometime after 100 C.E. (as much as 2,000 years later) largely as a social and political response to the rising influence of Buddhism in China. Philosophical Taoism is based on an understanding of an intelligence or force known as Tao (sometimes spelled Dao). The word Tao expresses a way or path. The Japanese version is Do, as in karate-do (the way of the empty hand) and bu-do (the way of war).

A number of celebrated Taoists authors have attempted to illuminate the Tao. An early one was King Wen of Zhou (one of the early states in the region before China existed as a nation). Around 1100 B.C.E. he allegedly penned the *I-Ching* (Book of Changes), a detailed description of the forces and processes of nature. Two others who lived perhaps 600 years later were Chuang Tzu, famous for penetrating Taoist stories, and Lieh Tzu, known for wise commentary.

The most famous Taoist author is the aforementioned semi-mythical figure named Lao Tzu, who has been so immortalized in myth and legend (some say he was born wise, white-haired, and bearded after gestating for 100 years in his mother's womb) that his role in the popular imagination is more relevant and important than whether or not he was a real person. If he was, he may have worked as a fortuneteller to the king of the Eastern Zhou dynasty during the sixth century B.C.E.

Fortunetellers in those days didn't play with crystal balls or cards. Nor did they make educated guesses based on subtle cues a customer unwittingly offered. Instead, they interpreted natural signs and forces. Having meditated for many years and cultivated great insight and sensitivity, a sage like Lao Tzu was able to predict both political cycles and the course of natural events such as storms and floods. His magnificent, maddening, and beautiful little book *Tao Te Ching* has been translated into more languages than any book save the Bible. It expresses the way the world works and the way the wise person lives in fewer than 5,000 brilliant, sometimes abstruse words. There may be no system of movement anywhere that is a purer expression of an underlying philosophy than tai chi is of Lao Tzu's Taoist philosophy.

Unlike some Western concepts of God, the Tao is not separate from people or from any other aspect of nature. Voiceless and disembodied, it proceeds indifferently, like the ocean tide. All-inclusive, omnipresent, omnipotent, and transcendent, it is nonetheless ineffable and unknowable. Fish don't sense the water in which they swim, and people—evolutionarily preoccupied by material survival and more recently psychosocially blinded by a culture of speed and greed—live behind a veil that won't allow them to perceive the Tao. Lifting this veil requires coming solidly into our body and quieting our mind. Tai chi practice helps us do both. There is no inherent conflict whatsoever between the physical practice of tai chi and any belief system or religion. It is often true, however, that after many years devoted practitioners often come to see spiritual matters differently.

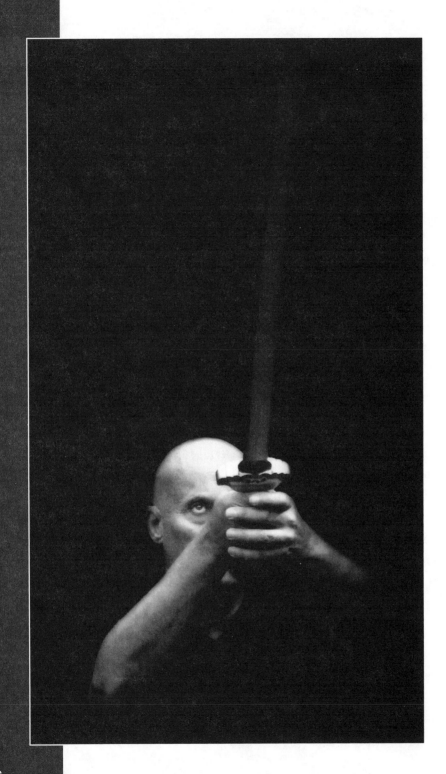

> I am like an idiot, my mind is so empty.
>
> TAO TE CHING, V.20 (STEPHEN MITCHELL, TRANSLATOR)

4

THE TAI CHI MIND

ONE GOOD DEED GOES UNPUNISHED

A few years back, just before Christmas, I entered a Starbucks drive-thru line for a cup of tea on my way to teach a morning tai chi lesson. When my turn came I gave my order at the billboard menu and then waited patiently for the cars in front of me to proceed. To my surprise, I heard the loud blast of a car horn. Glancing in the rearview mirror I saw the driver behind me, apparently dissatisfied with the alignment between his lips and the order taker's microphone, gesture for me to move forward. When I did not immediately comply—there was nowhere to go—he shouted an insult at me.

The equanimity and calm I train for evaporated as adrenaline flooded my body. I reached for the door handle with the intention of sending the rude driver to the dentist. As I was about to open the door, it suddenly struck me that whatever was wrong with him was now wrong with me, too. An idea floated into my head. When I reached the drive-through window, I told the barista I'd like to buy the guy's coffee.

"But he's a total jerk."

"Bad days happen to the best of us," I answered. "Just add whatever he's having to my tab."

"A random act of kindness, eh?" she asked as she regarded me thoughtfully.

"I'm a tai chi teacher. We have a certain philosophy about keeping our equilibrium. You could say that we always have three choices—I like to call them three doors. Door number #1 is to meet force with force. After that guy honked, if I took door #1 I would have just gone and punched him. Door #2 means yielding."

"You mean giving up?"

"Right. I would have gone over to his car and apologized for not moving four inches to the bumper of the car in front of me and maybe asked if I could wash his windshield for him, or shine his shoes."

"Yuck."

"Right. So in tai chi we always look for door #3. In some ways that's what the art is all about. That door is different every time. It is a creative solution to the problem, and one whose primary goal is to keep our equilibrium. The term for that equilibrium is wuji."

"Well hold onto your wuji, then, because the man back there isn't just drinking coffee this morning; he's ordered breakfast for five people. The total is $54."

That gave me pause. I had only ten dollars in my pocket. Did I really need to go through with my plan now? It took only a moment to decide. I took out my credit card and handed it over.

"Wow. You're sure?"

"Do it," I said.

After I'd signed the charge slip, I drove away without a backward glance. I felt relaxed and content, if a little thinner in the wallet. I also felt that I was completely finished with the exchange and had no desire to meet the honker on the road, either to receive his thanks or more acrimony. Accordingly, I stayed off the main thoroughfare and took a series of back roads to the park for my class.

Teaching was rewarding that day. I seemed to be able to sense my students' needs clearly and to give them what they desired. In demonstrating, my body felt relaxed and my movements energetic. When I returned home later, it was with a feeling of satisfaction at having done a pretty good day's work. All that changed when I checked my answering machine and found it full of messages from Starbucks. Apparently, the manager there had tracked me down using my credit card information. Following her messages was a series of increasingly persistent calls from a local NBC news reporter. I called him back.

"I've been waiting for hours to talk to you," he told me.

"What's this all about?"

"I'd like to come to your house."

"My house? Why?"

"It's about what happened at Starbucks."

"Are you kidding me? I bought a guy a cup of coffee."

"You didn't just buy him coffee, you bought breakfast for five people."

"So what? Why don't you find a real news story?"

"You don't understand. After you did that for him, he did it for the next person and that person did it for the person behind him, and this chain of kindness has been going on for hours. Six hours later, it's still happening. That's what makes it a story. Now if I can't come to your house will you please come back down to Starbucks so you can explain to our viewers why you did what you did?"

Seeing the opportunity to share some tai chi philosophy, I agreed to meet him. When I did, I explained that I had just been trying to keep my cool, that there was a difference between a random act of consciousness and a random act of kindness. The story ran that evening, quickly going national and then spreading around the world. Within twenty-four hours I had received messages of appreciation from as far away as Australia.

One lesson is not only that we almost always have a chance to avoid conflict by finding that third door. Another is that small, stabilizing acts seem to have a great effect in an unstable world. The cynical quip about no good deed going unpunished is not only untrue, but it seems that many can appreciate even a tiny gesture. More than that, it points out that the greatest benefit of tai chi training, at least in terms of the global community, may be what it does for the mind.

CREATION, DUALITY, AND THE ETERNAL BALANCE OF THE WUJI MIND

The term wuji originates in the Taoist creation story, which is quite a simple one. It says that in the beginning, before there was anything, there was naught but a still and empty state called wuji. Ready to burst into all that is, wuji may have been empty but it was pregnant with infinite possibility. In a fashion strongly reminiscent of the Big Bang, wuji spontaneously gave rise to what the Chinese call the 10,000 things. These things (the material world in all its variety and diversity) are organized into relative states (binary pairs) called yin and yang. These words may be familiar. Among countless other qualities, yin usually refers to dark, moist, quiet, female, low, and soft, while yang usually refers to bright, dry, loud, male, high, and hard. The idea of yin and yang pervades tai chi, and the material world as well. Thinking about them led to advances in mathematics that changed the world. Without yin/yang theory, for example, we would not have computers, the Internet, or all the communication tools so many of us enjoy. When yin and yang interact in nature, they do so in an ever-shifting, harmonious way. The name for this harmonious interplay between opposing forces is tai chi.

We Westerners have our own ideas about duality. While they might have begun with God creating heaven and earth in the Bible, they were formalized by the seventeenth-century French philosopher Rene Descartes, who asserted that we have one finite but indivisible mind and one finite but divisible body. His misguided notion that our mind and body are wholly distinct was compelling at the time, but it has become the source of much misunderstanding in the world. It may be fun to watch a science fiction movie in which a giant brain floats in a jar of bubbling blue liquid while its thoughts roam the galaxy free of a physical body, but ancient Taoists and modern biologists alike know that in fact mind and body are one "mindbody."

Recognizing that our flesh can interact with the world (we can stub a toe), our mind can interact with the world (we can receive bad news), and that our flesh and brain communicate, it is not hard to believe that they can also influence each other. In fact, how we move and eat affects our state of mind, and what we think and feel affects our state of body. The degree to which this is true is exemplified by a new scientific discipline, epigenetics, which explores the link between our beliefs and emotions and the very structure and expression of our DNA. The dialog between body and brain is the reason so-called lifestyle diseases (arthritis, diabetes, heart disease, etc.) respond so well to nutritional and psychological counseling, and to mind/body practices like tai chi.

When our mindbody responds negatively, we experience the phenomenon of stress, the primary reason for doctor visits in our country. Stress requires a blending of what is outside us with what is inside us, a combination of a negative event and a negative reaction. When we experience stress, we lose our cool. A traditional tai chi curriculum helps us to get it back. It trains us to be quiet, powerful, and creative, responsive but non-reactive, free of plans and expectations and devoid of attachment to material things and internal feelings. When we are in such a harmonious state, we are excellent at negotiating and at avoiding conflicts. The practice debugs and sharpens our on-board communications system, alerting us to emotional and physical problems while they are still small and easily solved.

NO PLANS, NO ATTACHMENTS, NO GOALS

Many years ago, my teacher's teacher, Chen Quanzhong, visited the United States from Xi'an, China. While he was here, he stayed in my home and we took photos together and ate meals. As I have no Chinese and he has no English, we communicated in gestures and smiles. Halfway through his visit my teacher, Master Yan, arranged for him to watch me perform some tai chi. I use the word perform advisedly, because I was so nervous. It was difficult to relax and maintain my wuji while being watched by the man who is arguably the greatest living practitioner of the art.

After botching a rendition of the tai chi straight sword by forgetting the moves halfway through and muttering a curse that brought me a warning look from my teacher, I was asked to spar and show the Grandmaster what I could do. To show me off to best advantage, my teacher picked one of my kung fu brothers in the school, a man much larger and stronger than I am, and we sparred for several rounds. I had more training and did well, but each time I triumphed I saw my Grandmaster shake his head sadly. I redoubled my efforts for the next round, but even though I bested my partner again and again, I received nothing but looks of dismay if not disgust.

Finally and totally demoralized, I approached my teachers, who were sitting together on chairs, arms folded, with serious looks on their faces.

"What did I do wrong?" I asked, chastened.

The Grandmaster pursed his lips and shook his head and said, "Noooooo."

Lacking many other English words, he used inflection, duration, and facial expression to achieve an entire lexicon around this single word. Seeing my struggle to divine his meaning my teacher broke in.

"You had a plan," he said.

"A plan? What do you mean? I beat him every round."

"Yes, but you might not have."

"I might not have, but I did," I replied in frustration.

"You used tricks. You used speed. You used technique."

I stared, trying to imagine what could possibly be wrong with those things. The Grandmaster interrupted, and my teacher listened to him intently. When he finished, I received the translation.

"Each time you fought, you saw things your partner was doing and you figured out ways to beat him," my teacher explained.

"And?" I answered, now totally exasperated.

"When your opponent changes his strategy, your plan may not work," my teacher said sternly. "The wuji mind moves the body purely, responding to each and every development as it arises. It is in the moment that you pause that your opponent can strike, the moment that you strategize that he can deceive you."

"But winning is a plan!" I cried.

"No. Winning is a goal, like survival. Big-picture goals allow you to move like water, able to respond to changes without attachment or restriction when things don't go your way or the unexpected happens; by contrast a plan is structured and set. The Grandmaster is not interested in seeing you apply the skills you bring from other arts you've learned. Rather than seeing ego, rigidity, ambition, and attachment to outcome, he wants to see your wuji mind and your flowing body."

Tai chi sets a very high philosophical and physical standard. While some martial arts are all about fighting in a cage in front of screaming fans or about surviving a firefight in a far-off land, tai chi trains us to flow in the face of whatever life dishes out. Moving like water and curating a mind empty yet pregnant with infinite possibility, tai chi may lead us to respond to an irate driver by buying his coffee, answer the gentle lover with our own brand of comfort, meet speed with what appears to be slowness but is actually perfectly anticipated positioning, and counter brightness with shadow at just the right angle to bring out all available intricacy and depth.

Tai chi is the perfect exercise because it creates harmony in the mindbody. It teaches spontaneity over strategy, suppleness over rigidity, joy over expectation, and acceptance over judgment. It trains us to go higher when our opponent goes up, lower when he goes down. The wuji mind challenges the event-based view of the universe Western science has given us, allowing us to see hurricanes, wars, plagues, flood, break-ups, firings, and punches not as isolated constructs of human experience, but as expressions of cycles in a dynamic, ever-changing world. It helps us to respond to such events without attachment or striving, without much effort but with maximal efficiency and effect. Tai chi practice, physically nuanced and mentally profound, trains us to balance the yin and the yang forces in every moment of every day, and in doing so create our own harmonious world.

THE MIND YOU BRING TO CLASS (AND HOW TO EAT HUMBLE PIE)

There is a great Zen parable about a student who comes to a famous master in search of the teachings. Rather than asking the master questions, however, the student spends some time talking about himself and how much he knows. As he drones on, the master heats some water for tea, and then serves it. He fills the student's cup, but after the cup is full he keeps on pouring. The tea goes all over the table and then all over the floor. The student leaps up in protest, only to hear the master tell him that like the cup, he is already too full of himself and his own ideas to accept new ideas.

After sixteen years of training in a wide range of Asian martial arts, I was teaching in a South Florida health club when a student gave me a piece of paper with a telephone number on it, telling me that some tai chi player had just come from China and was supposed to be pretty good. I called the guy, met him for breakfast, and spent the whole meal telling him how great I was. As I talked, he just chewed and nodded. Afterward, he suggested we spar outside. It was raining. We positioned ourselves, but the minute we touched, I fell down. "Slippery sidewalk," I said. We touched hands again. Wham. My tailbone hit the ground. I leapt up, brushed myself off, and grinned stupidly at him. "Must be my shoes," I said. We touched hands again. This time I went down a bit harder, and as I came up I desperately tried to figure out what it was he had done to me, and how I could possibly counter it. There was nothing for me. Not the slightest hint of information. I had not seen or felt anything at all. "Listen," I began. "Forget what I told you at breakfast. You obviously know things I need to learn. Would you teach me?"

In response, he turned around waved his hand in the air without looking at me. "You know everything already," he said, walking away.

Driving home, I cursed my own arrogance and resolved to change his mind. The next morning I took a paperback and a thermos and camped outside his front door. He saw me, ignored me, and went on his way. We repeated this scenario every morning for two weeks until he finally relented and agreed to teach me.

The next morning we met at a nearby park, where he instructed me to stand still with my arms out in front, eyes closed, not moving and not speaking. I did so for an hour while he drank tea at a picnic table and read a newspaper. I had never stood in one place that long and a fire burned in my arms, legs, shoulders, and disquieted mind. All the same, he had told me not to move and I was resolved to obey. After an hour I paid him for the lesson and we agreed to meet again later that week.

Three months passed, and three times a week I stood in agony while he drank tea and I tried to calm my thoughts. At the end of those months, he began to teach me movements, but, as I came to realize, he had been teaching me tai chi all along. The lessons had been difficult. Emptying my cup meant abandoning my ego as best I could, and letting go of as much bitterness, anger, humiliation, fear, judgment, and frustration as possible. In the end it was not just my legs that grew stronger, but my mind as well. I struggled with the process but something inside me had made me acquiesce to the deeper understanding that I was being offered. Perhaps it was realizing that the other way, to continue along the path of my self-congratulatory ignorance, would never lead to skill, satisfaction, or fulfillment.

Some of us come to tai chi looking for optimum health and have no idea it is even a martial art. Others come with a closet full of black belts behind them, searching for a way to deepen our understanding of energy, internal training, body mechanics, combat and philosophy. Whether we want to defend ourselves against the degenerative diseases of aging, parking lot thugs, or the restrictions of our own untamed mind, if we can empty our cup, tai chi will do for us what we want it to do.

TAI CHI AND ENLIGHTENMENT

Because tai chi is a path as well as a practice, the dividends are constantly unfolding. Cliché though it may be to say, it's about the journey as well as the destination. Still, and for all that, what might the destination be? What might we hope to gain if we really get into it and really practice patiently, diligently, and persistently? Certainly our health will improve. So will our energy, vitality, and sexual performance. We will come to confidently handle verbal and physical conflicts. In time, we may reach such a delightful state of equanimity and insight that we experience the world as a rush of marvels.

There is a word for this state of being, and the word is enlightenment. The very term suggests luminosity, clarity, and the opposite of darkness. It conjures fantasy and speculation, perhaps because those who know what it really is don't try to describe the indescribable. What we may say is that enlightenment, like genius, connotes experiencing all the usual things, but differently. An old Zen saying makes the point that before enlightenment, we go through our day doing the normal chores like chopping wood and carrying water, and after enlightenment, we do the same. To this description, the great Zen master, D.T. Suzuki, adds that when we are enlightened, we do all that we did before, but we do it two inches off the ground.

Enlightenment is not attached to any religion. It exists independent of any particular beliefs or faith. Because it is a state of mind (maybe a state of brain), if we can connect it to anything, it would be to psychology, or better, to neurobiology. In tai chi terms, an enlightened person lives in perfect harmony with nature, not having created the required perfect balance between yin and yang but having found it. The potential for enlightenment exists in all of us—we "merely" have to free ourselves from those things that keep us from it. The tai chi path to enlightenment begins with physical lessons that teach us to redirect force when it hits us, thereby keeping our emotional and physical balance.

There is great joy in being on such an exciting path. As our understanding grows, we become ever freer to change directions as water would, to flow easily and gracefully from one level of understanding to the next. The tai chi journey, always a challenge to our perseverance, creativity, discipline, and patience, is full of wonderful twists and turns. One thing is for sure. As we experience the growth from the martial exercise of tai chi ch'uan to the spiritual exercise of tai chi, we grow in unfathomable ways.

EXPLORATIONS

Science calls wuji homeostasis: a range within which we find physiological ease. In homeostasis, heart and respiratory rates are neither too fast nor too slow, and the level of hydration, nutrients, and circulating chemicals in our blood are at, or near, optimal levels. In homeostasis all our body systems are working as intended and we are emotionally and energetically stable. To maintain homeostasis we eat when we are hungry, drink when you are thirsty, rest when we are tired, stretch when we are stiff, calm ourselves when we are overwrought, relax when we are stressed, soothe ourselves when we are angry, and reassure ourselves when we are afraid. This set of explorations employs creative visualization—a useful training tool in any athletic endeavor— to explore the acute, immediate loss of wuji and how to use tai chi principles to restore it.

EXPLORATION #1

The Effects of Strong Negative Emotions

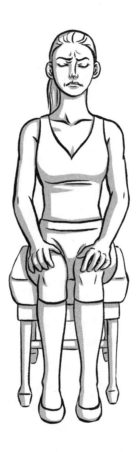

SITTING IN A COMFORTABLE STRAIGHT-BACKED CHAIR, CLOSE your eyes and visit the theater of your mind. Imagine that you are contentedly driving a car, minding your own business, your muscles relaxed. Suddenly, someone cuts you off. You slam on the brakes, narrowly escaping injury. Stopped in the middle of the road, the other driver lowers his window, lifts his middle finger, and shouts insults.

Feel your stress response build. Feel how your heart races and your adrenal glands squeeze. Feel your muscles tense and the prick of sweat on your hands and feet. Feel your breathing quicken and your belly roil. Cultivate this stress response, feeding it like a pet, grooming it and encouraging it so as to prolong the feeling and give you time to really explore it.

Focus on any righteous indignation you may feel, on any associations, outrage, or feelings of suffering an injustice. Notice any angry or retributive thoughts. Notice if any memories of previous violent confrontations arise. If they do, notice what physical manifestations you feel. In this deliberately controlled setting, take the time to become as familiar as possible with all aspects of your stress response. Once you have done so, you are ready for the next exercise.

EXPLORATION #2

Returning to
Emotional Equilibrium

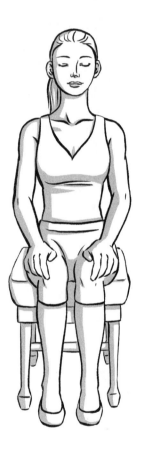

BEGIN AGAIN IN A COMFORTABLE, STRAIGHT-BACKED CHAIR, your body supported and relaxed. Imagine a string drawing our crown point up to heaven as you again visit the theater of the mind. Once more, imagine driving happily along in your favorite car. This time, however, see yourself in stormy weather and in a different geographic location. Beside you in the front seat is a loved one: a child, parent, or partner. This time, a vehicle comes out of the gloom, runs a traffic light, and heads straight for you. In a miraculous last-minute maneuver, you avoid a collision. The risk to someone beside you redoubles your outrage and you feel an even stronger rush of emotions than those that took you in the previous exploration.

Rather than embracing the feelings, this time you want to counter and control them. Breathe slowly and deeply. After a few minutes, notice your mind beginning to settle. Conjure an image of the reckless driver and see if you can't feel compassion for her. Imagine her in her boss's office being cruelly and unjustly fired. Watch as she is accompanied to his desk by security personnel, where—dejected and anxious about how she will ever meet her commitments and feed her kids—she collects her belongings. Imagine how she must feel as she carries them out of the building to the very same car that will soon take her careening into your car.

If you are able to run this movie in your head long enough, you might see her worrying about breaking the news to her family. Perhaps you can viscerally feel her state of mind as she runs the traffic light that very nearly brings her into disastrous contact with you. You might follow your imaginary progress past the near miss and actually envision the family interlude, the tears, the remonstrations, the desperation. Humanizing your "movie villain" not only replaces your rage with understanding and compassion but also generates a feeling of kinship with others and the larger world. While there are other techniques for assuaging anger and balancing negative feelings, this kind of visualization—when combined with a meditative posture and breath control—is the one most characteristic of tai chi.

EXPLORATION #3

Physically Opening the Third Door

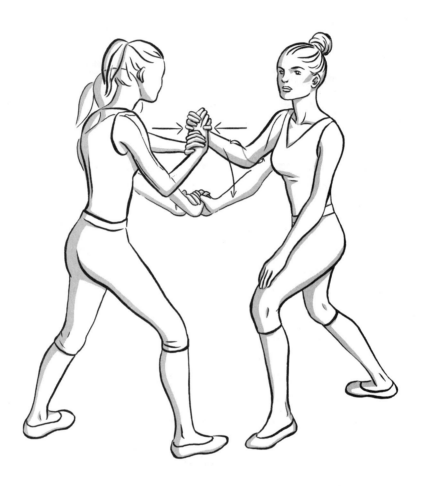

ALTHOUGH MANY PRACTITIONERS NEVER TEST OR APPLY THEIR physical mastery of the art, traditional tai chi training has us first repeating short movements as so-called solo exercises, next learning sequences of movements called forms, and finally working with a partner to increase our level of understanding. This third level of exploration ties visualization to the physical world.

To begin, choose a reliable partner who brings neither aggressiveness nor strong ego to the interaction, but instead is eager to assist. Facing each other at arm's length, assume a stance with right legs back and left legs forward, hips and shoulders square to each other, and feet slightly less than shoulder-width apart. Soften your knees, drop your lower back, keep a straight spine, and keep your shoulders down. Put your right hand against your partner's. Left hands are at rest.

Rooting as you learned to do in Chapter 2, ask her to push on you, and feeling her force, push back. If you can successfully transmit force to the ground, you should feel the pressure in your feet. In a contest of force, the stronger partner always prevails. If you are stronger, you might notice feelings of satisfaction, superiority, or even compassion for your partner. If you are the weaker partner, you may notice feelings of failure or frustration. Accept those feelings and proceed to the next step, which is to voluntarily yield. Notice how when you do, your partner's force immediately overcomes you, destroying whatever alignment you have attained and causing you to lose your balance. Surrender is emotionally and physically risky, leading to feelings of helplessness, righteous indignation, resentment or anger as well as the chance of injury.

In the last phase of this exploration, see if you can find a way to creatively redirect your partner's force. Start by turning your waist while keeping your elbow pointed inward and down. Now relax your chest, let your hips swivel, and drop down into your legs in order to bring your partner's hand downward and inward, helping her to lose her balance. Once you get the hang of this, switch roles and see if she can do the same to your push. The more nuanced your three-dimensional responses become, the more effective at meeting a variety of attacks you will be. Note that in these three exercises we have now gone from simply experiencing a loss of mental equilibrium to actually restoring both physical alignment and a clear, balanced mind.

Voices in Our Head

The term tai chi denotes a world organized into a binary interplay of opposites such as light and dark, male and female, good and evil, slow and fast, and more. Western science is growing ever more greatly into accord with a worldview of binary opposites. Even in quantum physics every particle is matched to an anti-particle. More, in exploring non-local phenomenon (currently-inexplicable forces that exist independent of time and distance) it was recently revealed that the spin of a photon (a unit of light energy) in one location determined the spin of a partner photon on the other side of the world, despite there being no understandable, material connection between the two.

On a far simpler and more concrete level, every one of us experiences life's binary choices from moment to moment. Should we stop or go; turn left or right; choose this relationship or that; this job or the other; the burger or the salad? When competing external forces create competing internal urges, we experience stress: "I really need to go to the gym, but I should spend the time with the kids; I know my boss expects this report by tonight, but if I stare at this screen for one more moment, my eyes are going to fall out of my head; I owe it to my sister to be loyal, but I really need to tell someone what she did."

Even when it comes to our tai chi practice, we may hear conflicting voices in our head. One voice may say: "Oh yes, this is good for me, ah, my body feels great, keep going, sink deeper, breathe evenly, move with more flow, hurts so good, makes me powerful," while another voice counters: "Tai chi moves don't puff up my arms like weight machines do; if I want to work out I should get back to the gym. This mindful tai chi practice is just a bunch of Chinese hooey. If I want to reduce my blood pressure I should just take a pill; if I want to defend myself, I should get a gun or pepper spray."

Tai chi is all about bringing opposing forces into harmonious balance. When one leg is heavy, the other is often light; when one hand is forward, the other is often back; when we shift weight, we make sure and keep both feet in connection with the ground. When we apply force in one direction, we make sure and counter by relaxing and sinking into the ground in the opposite direction. Tai chi puts a mental finger to our lips. We cannot be thinking about problems at the office when our mind is in the position of our fingers or toes. Our body cannot relax fully and deeply when our mind is full of anxious noise. The more we practice, the quieter and more integrated our mind becomes. Emotional poise comes with that integration, and grace, clear thinking and physical power do, too. It may not be easy and it may not be quick, but tai chi practice quiets those voices in our head.

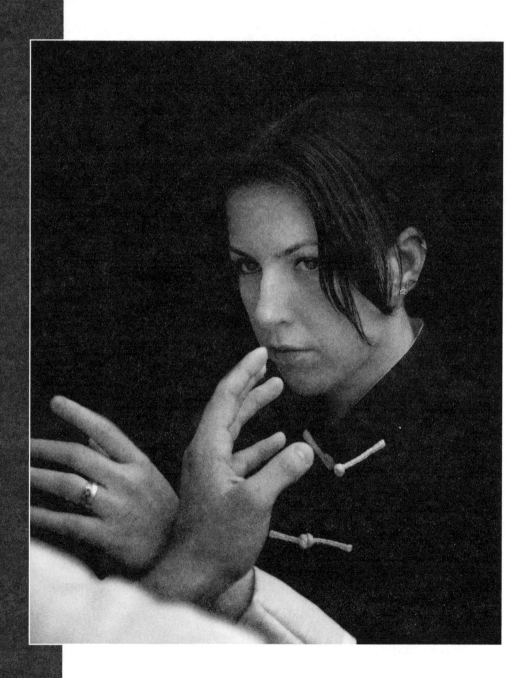

5

"In carrying about your more spiritual and more physical aspects
And embracing their oneness,
Are you able to keep them from separating?
In concentrating your qi and making it pliant,
Are you able to become the newborn babe?"

TAO TE CHING, V.10 (AMES AND HALL, TRANSLATORS)

QI, BREATH, AND QIGONG

WHAT IS QI?

This chapter explores a force beyond muscle power that is essential to the practice of tai chi. This energetic phenomenon has been recognized since the dawn of history and given different names around the world. Maori people refer to it as mana, the Greeks called it pneuma, the Japanese call it ki, yogis know it as prana, devout Christians might think of it as the Holy Ghost, some spiritually-minded scientists allow that it might be some ineffable force that lends atoms awareness of themselves, and tai chi players know it as qi (pronounced "chee").

In Chinese culture qi is a vibrant energy that seeps into so many aspects of life that it truly qualifies as one of the key concepts Chinese people use to make sense of the world. It appears in everyday language—your qi looks good today—and meanders like a nourishing stream through Chinese literature, fine arts, music, science, and philosophy. Qi is a key concept in the study of tai chi because it is also the root currency of Traditional Chinese Medicine—one of the three legs of the tai chi tripod. The TCM practitioner manipulates several different types of qi in managing health and disease. First is the primordial qi that arises at the union of sperm and egg. Next is the daily qi nourished by what we eat and drink and how we breathe and move. There is also surface qi (wei qi) that guards us against invading pathogens, and the various forms of qi unique to different organs and bodily systems (liver qi, heart qi, digestive qi, etc.).

Like life, evolution, and other sophisticated concepts, the phenomenon of qi conjures different images and associations for each of us. To some people, it is an ineffable force. To others, it is a purely physical sensation. Advanced martial artists and healers find qi a clearly discernable energy that can be cultivated, manipulated, and even transmitted. Precisely because it is so multidimensional, qi has been hard for Western investigators to isolate and identify in the laboratory. Hotly pursuing the subject, some believe that it may be light energy, blood, lymph, heat, or the electrical potential across cell membranes. Others suspect that qi might be ultra-low frequency sound or even a function of the vibration of quantum "strings" or sub-atomic particles, and therefore a feature of the quantum universe.

The early Taoist assertion that the universe is pervaded by qi matches the very latest in astronomical discoveries, which point to the existence of all-pervasive, so-called "dark" energy and "dark" matter. Modern-day Taoist feng shui masters still design and arrange homes and businesses in accordance with the flow of qi just the way they did millennia ago. They still see qi as earth energy whose flow, when properly regulated and encouraged, makes for positive results such as health, happiness, and prosperity but when ignored or misused results in a living or working space that can lead to stagnant creativity, illness, and misery.

The good news is that most tai chi players experience qi directly, and without any need for scientific validation. Those of us who already feel, sense, and know qi have good cues as to how to enhance rather than deplete it, encourage its free flow rather than obstruct it, and draw upon it to enjoy life more fully. We may discern it as a familiar tingling in our hands or the ability to practice harder, longer, and in deeper stances. We may feel it as the energy that keeps us going, rejuvenates our sexual performance, allows us to bounce back after exercise, and keeps us alert and awake even after a long, sleepless, airplane journey. We may construe it as enthusiasm, youthful vigor, resistance to falling ill, or the quality that steers us toward certain people and away from others. We may also know it as the energizing quality of a certain color, food, sound, or scent.

Whether we realize it or not, we are always sensing qi in the people around us, and in our surroundings. If we have ever said, "I just feel so good when I'm in that house," or "I just love her energy," or "I don't know why, but when that complete stranger walked into the room, I just had the sense he was creepy," we have unconsciously responded to qi. Could it be that qi manifests as pheromones, a smell, or a subconscious association with someone or something in our past? It could, but even so it falls under the umbrella of the energy of life. In a nuts-and-bolts way we can say that when we wake up well rested and full of energy we have strong qi, and when we are depleted, exhausted, poisoned by indulgence, or ill, our qi is weaker. We can also sometimes feel when the qi flow to some particular body part or organ is stagnant or blocked, such as when we have a sore knee or aching stomach. In the end it is not a matter of whether qi is actually there, but rather if we are aware of it. Those of us who do not yet recognize qi have only to start practicing tai chi to wake up this particular sensibility.

QI FLOW IN THE BODY

At the union of our father's sperm and our mother's egg, what some call our "primordial" qi was created. We can think of this as the principal in our qi bank account. Over time, it slowly draws down until the last moment of the last day of our life, when the balance falls to zero. From a Taoist point of view there is only one way to grow this principal and that is to meditate. We can draw interest from the principal, however, and tai chi practice helps us to invest this principal well by distributing it throughout the body in a bid for a long, healthy, pain-free life.

Although many Taoist practitioners are fond of directing the flow of qi using their intention, the traditional tai chi player understands that qi flow in the body is a sublime and balanced process that has developed over millions of years of human evolution. It is unlikely that any practitioner, no matter how accomplished, knows better than nature does where his or her qi should flow. Accordingly, and in contradiction to many qigong masters who see things differently, in tai chi we want only to relax the body, remove obstructions and limitations, and allow the qi to flow unguided where and when it needs to in order to bring us optimal vitality and health. Tai chi relaxation, sung, is designed to encourage the flow of qi through and along routes identified by Traditional Chinese Medicine. It's worth a look at the details of these routes, if only to develop an appreciation for the detail and holistic aspects of the medical system that underpins tai chi.

The major routes for qi flow are the eight so-called extraordinary vessels and twelve standard meridians or pathways. While qi does not always behave as a simple fluid might, it is reasonable to think of these channels as pipelines. Along these pathways there are hundreds (if not more) therapeutically important points. The eight extraordinary vessels maintain homeostasis (keep the body running the way it prefers to) and are also known as psychic channels. Some of them coincide with the standard meridians, and all of them form an interconnected web of qi flow. One circles the waist, another penetrates from the front to the back of the body, and others run along the legs. The most important ones are the Governing (Du) and Conception (Ren) Vessels, which run up the midline of the back and down the front of the body respectively. These two are involved in the so-called Greater and Lesser Heavenly Circles, the primary paths of overall energy circulation in the body and a subject we will consider in some detail in the chapter on tai chi meditation.

The twelve meridians represent the interaction between yin (soft, female, winter, cold, slow, dark) and yang (hard, male, summer, hot, fast, bright) energy in the body. In the healthy person there is a perfect balance. Each meridian is also associated with a time of day, a personal quality, and an emotion—the theory being that as qi flows through the body it does so in accordance with cycles and forces both inside the body and outside in the world. As such, each meridian has a connection to a function of our character and role in the world.

Because TCM is an observation-based system, there is also a correlation between each meridian and the five elements of the Taoist cosmology (earth, water, fire, metal, and wood) that comprise our world. In each meridian, energy flows either toward the center of the body (centripetal direction) or away from it (centrifugal direction). The major therapeutic acupuncture points are found along these meridians, as are the points most important to tai chi relaxation. Again, details of the pathways differ a bit, but here is a basic overview:

The Lung Meridian is primarily yin and related to metal. Energy flows through it in a centrifugal direction across the top of the chest at the base of the shoulders and out each arm to the base of the thumbnail. This meridian is most active from 3:00–5:00 a.m. and is associated with grief and intolerance. Considered a source of self-esteem and connection with the pure qi of the world around us, this meridian is connected to our spiritual dimension.

The Large Intestine Meridian is primarily yang and related to metal. Energy flows through it in a centripetal direction from the base of the nail of the index finger up along the arm to the shoulder and neck to the area of the nostril. This meridian is most active from 5:00–7:00 a.m. and is associated with guilt. The work of letting go of what we do not need is the province of this meridian, which is in charge of the body's waste system.

The **Stomach Meridian** is primarily yin and related to earth. Energy flows through it in a centrifugal direction from beneath the eye, down the chest and abdomen to the front of the leg to end at the base of the second toenail. This meridian is most active from 7:00–9:00 a.m. and is associated with greed and disgust. It affects our ability to integrate information and accept love.

The **Spleen Meridian** is primarily yin and related to earth. Energy flows through it in a centripetal direction from the base of the nail of the big toe along the inside of the leg to the side of the torso to end below the armpit. This meridian is most active from 9:00–11:00 a.m. and is associated with anxiety and concern about the future. In TCM the spleen is involved with extracting energy from food, so this meridian also affects our ability to concentrate strongly and think clearly.

The **Heart Meridian** is primarily yin and related to fire. Energy flows through it in a centrifugal direction from under the armpit down the inner side of the arm to the base of the smallest finger. This meridian is most active from 11:00 a.m.–1:00 p.m. and is associated with the strong emotions of both joy and anger. Because the heart is a quintessential organ, this meridian affects the functioning of the other meridians in the body.

The **Small Intestine Meridian** is primarily yang and related to fire. Energy flows through it in a centripetal direction from the base of the little fingernail up the arm to the side of the neck, then around to the front of the face and back over to the front of the ear. This meridian is most active from 1:00–3:00 p.m. and is associated with sadness and insecurity. This meridian helps us to stay clear by sorting out good and bad, pure and impure in our lives.

The **Bladder Meridian** is primarily yang and related to water. Energy flows through it in a centrifugal direction beginning at the inside corner of the eye, then going up and over the top of the skull then down the back near the spine before splitting to go down the back of the legs to end at the base of the nail of the smallest toe. This meridian is most active from 3:00–5:00 p.m. and is associated with impatience and restlessness. It is the energetic pathway along which residual energy is stored, and thus helps us to fight fatigue.

The Kidney Meridian is primarily yin and related to water. Energy moves through it in a centripetal direction from the middle of the front part of the ball of the foot up the inside of the leg to just above the genitals, then along the chest before ending between the collarbone and the first rib. This meridian is most active from 5:00–7:00 p.m. and is associated with fear and indecisiveness. It helps us to have resolve and a sense of purpose, and drives us to get things done.

The Pericardium Meridian is primarily yin and related to fire. Energy flows through it in a centrifugal direction beginning on the chest and then down the arm and hand to the base of the middle fingernail. This meridian is most active from 7:00–9:00 p.m. and is associated with emotional hurt, jealousy, and regret, and it protects us from shock and hurt.

The Triple Burner Meridian is primarily yang and related to fire. Energy moves through it in a centrifugal direction from the outside edge of the ring finger up the hand and arm to the head, ending just below the eyebrow. This meridian is most active from 9:00–11:00 p.m. and is associated with depression and despair. It regulates both physical and emotional warmth.

The Gall Bladder Meridian is primarily yang and related to wood. Energy moves through it in a centrifugal direction from the outside corner of the eye across the head and down the side of the body and leg to end at the fourth toe. This meridian is most active from 11:00 p.m.–1:00 a.m. and is associated with strong anger and rage. It affects vision, judgment, and optimism.

The Liver Meridian is primarily yin and related to wood. Energy moves through it in a centripetal direction from the large toenail up the leg and across the belly to the chest. This meridian is most active from 1:00–3:00 a.m. and is associated with unhappiness and also with abiding anger. It affects our ability to plan and execute life strategies.

TAI CHI BREATHING

Our lungs are like balloons hanging inside our chest cavity. Filling and emptying them is accomplished by changing the pressure outside of them relative to the pressure inside. If the pressure in the chest cavity is greater than it is inside the lungs, air moves out and we exhale. If the pressure in the chest cavity is less than it is inside the lungs, air moves in and we inhale. Various breathing techniques are no more or less than the use of the muscles of the torso and abdomen to effect the way we change the pressure in the chest cavity.

How we breathe affects how we use and distribute our qi. When we are infants, we have all the energy (a TCM practitioner would say all the lung qi) we need to cry and cry without going hoarse or losing our breath. As we get older, despite having bigger and more developed lungs, we seem never to have that kind of vocal energy again. Only if we train to sing opera or have a special gift can we hope to achieve, with great diligence and practice, what came to us so effortlessly when we were babies.

One reason this is true is that babies instinctively channel everything to the vocal muscles while relaxing the rest of the body completely. Another reason is that babies breathe with the diaphragm and muscles of the lower body rather than with the muscles of the chest. Later in life, we abandon this practice and start using chest muscles— particularly those between the ribs—as a response to stress. Essentially, using our chest muscles is a form of wincing, which happens because we tense up, not down.

We can think of the human body as a bag of water suspended from sticks we call bones. They are special sticks, granted, with factories inside them and the properties of healing and rejuvenation, but they are sticks nonetheless. The bag of water is also full of fluids of varying densities, some more solid than others, but the whole contraption responds to being squeezed by the muscles that encase it. The largest and strongest of those muscles are down low in the body, including the gluteals, the quadriceps, the abdominals, the Iliacus, Psoas major, and more. The squeeze those muscles put on the body is therefore more forceful at bottom than top, and the body responds by bulging at the top like a water balloon seized from the bottom.

Feeling this bulging and tightness in our chest, we fight back and use our chest muscles to breathe. Unlike the diaphragm, which is made of smooth muscle and has evolved for repeated, rest-free use, the fibers in our chest muscles are striated. That means they get tired quickly. Breathing with the muscles in our chest leads to fatigue. A baby could never cry for hours on end if it used its chest muscles. If you watch a baby breathe, particularly when she is distressed, you will see her belly rapidly rising and falling while the chest seems barely to move at all. This so-called "belly breathing" is a typical skill developed in tai chi, meditation, and other mindfulness exercises.

As we have discussed, relaxation is the most critical component of tai chi practice, and there is a strong link between relaxation and breath. A long, slow exhale is almost automatically tied to a muscular "letting go"; inhaling, conversely, can create stress if done the wrong way. Remember that tai chi is typically performed as a series of movements linked together into what we call a form. The transitions between these movements often receive insufficient attention. What we do with these transitions is inhale through them and then exhale when performing the next move or posture. This general guideline becomes a bit challenging when our movements are slow but our breathing is fast. This scenario is typical for beginners, as the movements demand much of muscles not yet trained and the relaxation that comes later and slows breathing down has not yet developed. Conversely, in advanced practice we find the paradox of explosive movements done rapidly while maintaining great softness and relaxation and slow, even breathing.

Until we have the tai chi experience of moving, meditating, and breathing as one, we should simply focus on allowing our breath to move as simply, easily, and as free of edges and pauses, as the tide on the beach. Like the yin/yang symbol of tai chi, wherein the two interlocking fish each bear an eye the color of the other, there should be a little bit of inhale in our exhale, and a little bit of exhale in our inhale. The idea of two streams moving simultaneously but in opposite directions gives us a sense of the smooth effortlessness of tai chi breathing.

WHAT IS QIGONG?

While tai chi has been greatly simplified and diluted over the years, even the most accessible versions of the art require correct alignment, memory of complex movements, relaxation, and eventually attention to breath. There is a way to get some of the same benefits albeit without the martial, spiritual, and philosophical aspects of the art, and that is to practice some form of qigong. The word qigong means energy work, and implies using the breath in combination with physical movement. Any movement work done with attention to energy can bear the qigong label. When practiced with no martial intent and with the goal solely of improving health, tai chi, despite its fighting roots, can be considered a type of qigong.

The energetic goal of qigong is the same as it is for tai chi, namely to use movements and breath to cultivate jing, the body's sexual fluid essence (more about this in the next chapter), convert it to qi, and thence to shen, a word that connotes an awakened spirit. These three elements, jing, qi, and shen, are the Holy Grail of all Taoist practices, and are known as the Three Treasures.

Because of the advantages it confers on the practitioner, qigong was long taught as a closed-door family secret known to both common and highborn people alike. These days, qigong is practiced by millions of (mostly older) people across Asia, but especially in China. Qigong is growing by leaps and bounds as a healing modality in the West, too. Based on either Taoist or Buddhist principles and often named for families or animals, there are literally thousands of different styles or systems of qigong. Amazingly, these healing "technologies" are so ancient that they are referenced in works going back many thousands of years. Some of them make a nice complement to tai chi practice, and can even serve as a warm-up to the main event.

One of the most popular qigong sets is The Eight Pieces of Brocade, which has been practiced so long that it is rendered very precisely on an amazingly preserved silk scroll discovered in Changsha, Hunan Province, China, and dated to 168 B.C.E. Many variants of its eight movements exist, but all activate the major energy pathways of our body and, over time, enhance health and longevity. We can enjoy this sequence of movements, described below, as many times a day as we wish, but must always remember to time our breath to coincide with the movement and to perform the set in the order presented. The sole exception is number five where the best idea is simply to let our breath flow as it will, without holding. The first seven movements should be repeated eight times in total, alternating sides where possible, always timing breath and movement to begin and end together. The last movement is traditionally done only seven times.

PUSH TO THE SKY: Standing with feet shoulder-width apart, knees slightly bent and lower back flat, we inhale as we raise our hands up the middle, gracefully over our head, palms up, fingertips pointing in toward each other. Keeping our shoulders down and relaxed as possible, we open our chest while avoiding shoulder tension. At the apex, we consciously relax and begin a slow exhale timed to bring our hands down the outside to meet by our navel, then go up again with the next breath.

THE ARCHER: In a wide, horse-riding stance and with hands in loose fists knuckles to knuckles in front of our breastbone, we inhale and look to the right, extending our right hand as if holding an archery bow and looking toward an imaginary target. At the same time we pull the left hand away while keeping the elbow crooked, fingers curled as if around a bowstring. As our hands separate, our chest opens and our shoulder blades pinch together. At the end of the inhaled breath and with the hands fully parted, we exhale and bring them back together. If our knee health and leg strength allows, we sink progressively deeper into our stance with each repetition.

TWIST WITH ARMS: We start with knees soft and feet together. Inhaling, we turn our body and look to the right as we stretch our left hand up as far as it will go while turning our fingertips inward, palm up as if pushing up against the ceiling. At the same time we stretch our right hand downward as if pushing on the floor, again turning our fingertips inward. After a robust stretch, we exhale, returning our hands to our sides and then repeat on the other side—this time with our left hand down and our right hand up. We are wringing the torso as if it were a towel with this movement, but our spine must stay perfectly straight: no leaning to the side, forward, or back.

TWIST WITHOUT ARMS: This exercise stretches the lower back and is identical to the previous except that the arms remain loosely by our side, emphasizing the spinal twist and the stretch we feel in our lower back. Because this is a simple movement it represents a good opportunity to coordinate the breath and turning.

TORSO CIRCLES: Starting with a wide stance and a flat, extended back, we bend down and forward as much as possible, pointing our chin at the ground before us. We circle our torso first clockwise four times and then counter-clockwise four times, concentrating on not losing our balance and letting our breath flow free and easily without worrying about coordinating it with the movements. As we reach back, we allow our hips to come forward for balance. If we feel dizzy, we concentrate on looking where we are going before we get there and following our eyes.

TOE TOUCH: Beginning with our feet shoulder-width apart and our hands high and open in an "I surrender" position, we inhale while arching our back and feeling a strong backward stretch, then we exhale and bend forward, keeping our knees slightly bent, and touch our fingertips to our toes, or as far down as we can manage. In this position we feel a gentle stretch in our back and hamstrings before rising to repeat.

DYNAMIC TENSING AND RELEASING: This exercise resembles a classic karate punch, with the hands in fists and punching in alternating fashion. Standing with our feet shoulder-width apart, we extend one hand while retracting the other. As we extend our fist forward to our front, we tense the entire body—from the toes to the fingers—including our face, which should be in a scary grimace, and our gluteals, abdomen, legs, and arms. We maintain this dynamic tension until our outgoing fist returns to its place at our hip, at which time we suddenly and thoroughly release all bodily tension until we are as soft as overcooked fettuccine. The most important part of this exercise is the moment when we go from maximally tense to maximally relaxed, for this trains us to be able to let go of physical tension in a deliberate and nearly instantaneous fashion.

SHAKE DOWN THE QI: This is the simplest exercise of the series. With knees slightly soft and feet touching we keep our back straight as we come up on our tiptoes on our inhaling breath, then suddenly drop, allowing the impact of our heels on the ground to knock the breath out of us in an exhale. For reasons of Chinese numerology and tradition, this is the only exercise in the series that we repeat seven times instead of eight, focusing on becoming more and more relaxed with each passing repetition.

STAYING ON A GOOD QIGONG PATH

Lao Tzu, the great sage whose wisdom is a foundation of Taoist practice, said that although his Way is a simple, straightforward path, most people inexplicably prefer to get lost on shortcuts or wandering around in the mountains. What he is trying to say is that there are a few simple guidelines to follow in order to live a balanced, rewarding life as free as possible from life's trials, but that many people choose not to follow them. Rather than engaging dogged persistence and self-discipline, some of us tend to give in to our whims, impulses, and urges.

Everyone experiences temptations in life, but in the world of qigong these can be especially seductive. Rather than leading us to a calm mind, a long, fulfilling life, and a healthy body, certain qigong practices, if indulged, can produce results that to non-practitioners seem the purview of fantasy novels or science fiction films. A short sample of these includes the alleged ability to sense and heal illness in others, see auras, bend a spear against our throat, walk on rice paper without tearing it, break stones with our bare hands, lie down on nails, walk on fire, push needles through panes of glass or wood, sit under a frigid waterfall, or exercise amazing breath control.

Such skills are not particularly rare among people who practice Taoist exercises, but in the context of modern American culture—with its emphasis and reliance upon technology over mind/body practice— they certainly seem outlandish. Fortunately, both tai chi and authentic qigong are more often and more relevantly used to produce solid, satisfying results that keep us on the path to clarity, health, and longevity.

Sensing Qi in Your Hands

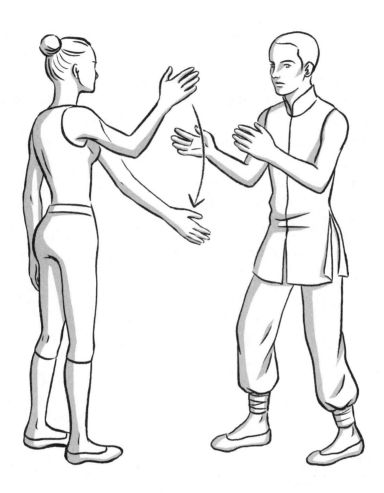

IN THIS EXPLORATION YOU WILL LEARN TO RECOGNIZE THE sensation of qi flow in your hands. To begin, stand in a relaxed pose with your feet shoulder-width apart and elbows and shoulders down and relaxed. Put your hands in front of you and rub them vigorously together until the friction brings heat. When you stop, you may feel a subtle, gauzy, presence between your palms. If not, repeat until you do.

Now draw the hands very slowly apart, inch-by-inch, while maintaining awareness of the fuzzy, electric, pins-and-needle ball of energy between them. The sensation diminishes as you move your hands apart. At some point you will no longer feel it, but after practicing tai chi or qigong for some months or years, you may be able to open your arms wide and still feel the energetic connection.

Once you've spent some time practicing, you can test your ability to sense your qi field by enlisting the aid of a partner. Standing with your eyes closed and your hands apart, concentrate on your qi field as your partner passes his or her hand between yours, interrupting the connection. This should be done silently and without hint or warning. Once you are able to reliably feel the hand passing through your field, you can feel confident you have improved your sensitivity to energy.

EXPLORATION #2

Belly Breathing

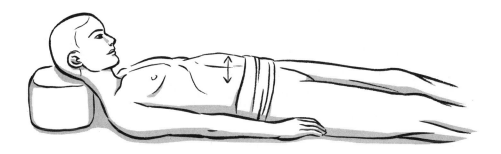

THE SINKING, RELAXING, SPIRALING MOVEMENTS OF TAI CHI
pump our qi through your body in much the way a bellows pumps air
to fan the flames in a fireplace. The bigger and deeper our movements,
the stronger the action of the bellows. The way we breathe can also
enhance this pumping, effectively pressurizing our qi flow.

The first of the two breathing exercises is belly breathing.

To breathe with your belly is to loosen your abdominal muscles
with your inhale and contract them upon exhale. To get the hang of
this, lie down on your back and use a thin pillow to lift your head so
you can look down at your belly and monitor your breath. Avoid using your chest to breathe, something we are all inclined to do. Noticing this tendency, consciously relax the muscles between the ribs and
soften the muscles of your chest until your whole upper body sinks
into the floor or bed and you feel a sense of pervasive calm.

Inhaling, watch the stomach rise; exhaling, watch the stomach fall.
The act of focusing on your breathing may cause you to breathe too
quickly and deeply at the start, so try to control your respiratory rate.
The breath should have the quality of the tide, moving in and moving

out without a perceptible stop or hold. You may wish to practice this for five or ten minutes.

While you do not want to consciously force the breath while you are moving in tai chi (especially at the beginning, awareness of your breath is very helpful. In particular, you can notice the relationship between breath and relaxation. It is natural to soften and sink your torso into your pelvis upon exhale, and worth trying not to tense up upon inhale. It is fine to inhale when transitioning from one posture or movement to the next, so long as you remain relaxed, and to exhale with the execution of a tai chi maneuver.

EXPLORATION #3

Reverse Breathing

SO-CALLED REVERSE BREATHING DEVELOPS NATURALLY AFTER some years of tai chi practice, but we can get a taste of it here. It is an especially effective way to "charge" you qi.

Remember, breathing techniques are a matter of using muscles to change the pressure in the chest cavity relative to the pressure in the lungs. As does belly breathing, reverse breathing requires that the chest and intercostal muscles be left out of the process and the work be accomplished with the diaphragm. This time, however, we use the muscles of the abdomen and back to assist the diaphragm in a different and opposite way than we did when belly breathing. To experiment with this, stand in a comfortable position with your arms by your sides and your feet shoulder-width apart. Inhaling, contract your abdomen gently; exhaling, let it loose. It may take a while to manage this coordination. Remember not to involve the chest at all. Inhaling you may feel the lower back around and above the tailbone (Ming Men or Heaven's Gate in Traditional Chinese Medicine) expand. You may also experience a sensation of fullness around the kidneys.

Because reverse breathing involves conscious contraction, and because it is in itself a powerful qi pump, you have to be rather careful with this exercise. Pumping too much can create imbalances and problems. The key here is to make this a gentle exploration. Don't force your breath. If you feel lightheaded, stop. Each inhale should be no more than half of our full capacity, and each exhale should be a matter of allowing the breath to leave the body rather than pushing it out. The result of five minutes or so of reverse breathing is that you will feel enlivened, energized, and awakened, but gently so.

Acupuncture

Due to tai chi's qualities of deep relaxation and turning, the practice does a great job of moving qi and stimulating acupuncture points. Sometimes, however, we need medical intervention that is swifter and less subtle than a simple round of form practice. Acupuncture is a healing modality of Traditional Chinese Medicine that has been successfully administered for many thousands of years, and one often relied upon by tai chi players in addition to—or in lieu of—Western therapies. Acupuncture manipulates the flow of energy, qi, through pathways called meridians. These pathways are also utilized in the medical practices of other Asian countries, and, in fact, have been found outlined on tattoos of a man frozen in a snowstorm in the European Alps some 5,000 years ago. This suggests that other cultures have long recognized the way energy flows through the body.[1]

A typical acupuncture treatment involves penetrating the skin with tiny needles, but some styles of acupuncture (Japanese toyohari, for instance) don't require such penetration. In China, the typical course of therapy seems to be treatments every day for ten days, a break, then another similar course if needed. On our shores it is more typical to go once or twice a week for a month or two before lasting results are achieved. Most sessions last fifteen to thirty minutes in a quiet room, during which the patient often falls asleep.

Without surgery or pharmaceuticals, acupuncture activates qi where it is stagnating or blocked, and helps it flow smoothly. Practitioners vary in their needling technique. In China, needles are long and thick and enthusiastically "rowed," as Chinese patients apparently expect discomfort and associate it with results. Citing the lower pain threshold of Americans, most acupuncturists on our shores use smaller gauge needles, but often still move them to elicit a "heavy" feeling. Most patients here don't seem to find the sessions particularly uncomfortable.

Acupuncture has been extensively studied and verified to be effective in chronic and acute conditions ranging from asthma and insomnia to pain, post-traumatic stress disorder, osteoarthritis, migraine headaches, fibromyalgia, and many more. It has also proven to be effective at enhancing fertility and immune system function while curbing appetite and addictions like smoking and drinking.

Its effectiveness has led some Western scientists to pejoratively ascribe acupuncture's healing powers to a "placebo effect," a term meaning "healing that takes place because we believe it will." As we learn more, this term is rapidly losing relevance, for it turns out that the body's ability to heal itself is incredibly powerful and desirable; perhaps even a new "gold standard" against which all treatment should be judged.

Pushed along by cultural and market forces, American medicine is evolving. Old prejudices are giving way to open minds. The new model of integrative medicine is patient centered and embraces any and all effective solutions to the patient's health problems. Even so, some folks, including older Western MDs, still talk about whether or not they "believe" in acupuncture. Such thinking is ill informed and outdated. One might as well speculate about whether to believe in aspirin, morphine, insulin, surgery, or an MRI. The question is not *whether* acupuncture works, but *how* it works, and whether it is the appropriate therapy for a particular syndrome, problem, symptom, disease, or patient.

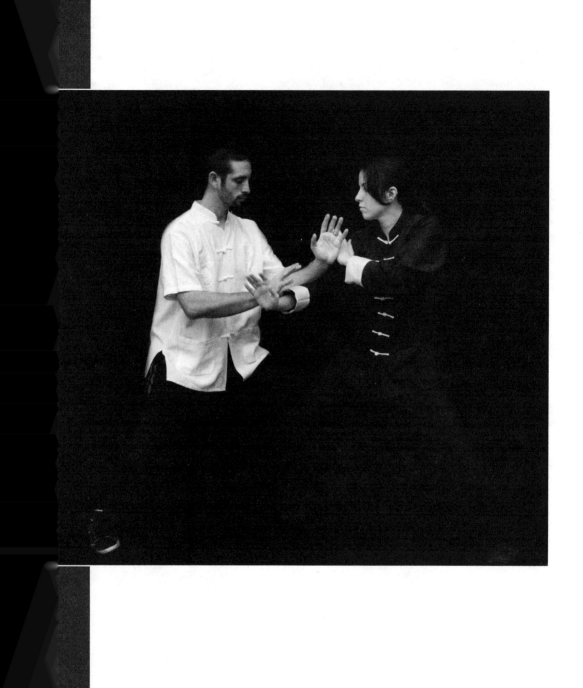

6

"One who respects the body equally with
all under heaven
may be entrusted with all under heaven.
One who cherishes the self equally with all under heaven
May be entrusted with the world."

TAO TE CHING, V.13 (SAM HAMILL TRANSLATOR)

SENSITIVITY, SENSUALITY, AND SEX

As seekers and questers we strive to find the beauty and the good in the world, and to avoid the traps that lead many others into a judgmental, negative state of constant conflict. Even so, we might unintentionally build emotional or physical walls to prevent people, and pain, from entering. While such protective strategies can be useful, they often persist long after they are needed, and take more effort than they bring joy. Tai chi practice helps us to shed these habits by encouraging us to draw on our passion, energy, and intelligence to create a harmonious interplay of opposing forces and allow us to live and love with greater satisfaction.

This wholeness is revealed by one of tai chi's most sought-after skills—sensitivity. Ardent tai chi players meditate to comprehend sensitivity, attend workshops to learn about it, and practice endlessly to cultivate it. Because tai chi is not only the perfect exercise but an art form that manifests on physical, philosophical, and spiritual levels, tai chi sensitivity is a multidimensional talent that bears on fighting prowess, emotional equilibrium, and our ability to sense internal and external changes. If we want to fully understand tai chi, we must become more sensitive.

WHAT IS TAI CHI SENSITIVITY?

The tai chi classics, scrolls written centuries ago, exhort us to arrive at our opponent's destination before he departs for it; even to know what he is going to do before he does it. In this context, sensitivity is a martial skill (ting jing in Chinese). It is all about touch, and the neurological cascade that follows it: how we acquire information and process it to maximum effect. There is always information to be gained by an opponent's attitude, energy, eyes, movements, and even smell, but deception—the good fighter's secret weapon—may lurk in some of that information. A good tai chi player will be able to sort things out at the first moment of physical contact. This means she will be able to feel the opponent's strategy—in which direction she is actually headed and to what purpose—and even how firm or shaky is her connection with the ground. Once the opponent's intention is clear, the tai chi player relies on rootedness and relaxation to follow the movement so as to gain and maintain the advantage.

Ting jing requires Taoist meditation, proper instruction and much practice. Seventeenth generation Chen family Grandmaster Chen Quanzhong (my teacher's teacher and sometimes mine) tells the story of Chen De Lu, one of his own teachers and a man of prodigious talents. Grandmaster Chen relates that Chen De Lu was able to interpret and react to pressure as light as that given by a small bird sitting on his hand after being lured in with a piece of fruit. Before the bird flapped its wings to fly off, it would ever so subtly shift in its stance and press down with its feet. At that moment, Chen would move ever so slightly downward so the bird would not be able to push off, effectively trapping it without grasping it. My Grandmaster tells me that Chen was even able to do this with a moth, whose infinitesimal weight and force would give up no information even to most other very advanced players.

Past masters achieved what they did because their lives depended upon it. Even though most of us are neither entrenched in a battlefield nor ever plagued by bandits, modern society is full of challenges to our well being, some of which are pernicious enough to cost us our lives. These include the degenerative diseases of aging, the demands of an increasingly competitive world, environmental sensitivities, genetic weaknesses, and all the modern weapons of mass distraction (the Internet, TV, movies, games, a deluge of news media) that vie for our attention.

To develop ting jing as our tai chi ancestors did means not believing everything we are told by people who have something to gain from us, establishing our own priorities, guarding our time more closely than we do our money, and guarding our energy most of all. It means limiting entertainments and distractions in favor of a practice brimming with mindful intent and focused on our own inner cycles and workings. If we do this, we will find ourselves capable of overcoming opponents by finding their center of balance with merely a touch. Our practice will also make us better listeners, able to apply sensitive listening to improving our performance and position at work, as well as cultivating compassion and heading off conflicts at home.

EAVESDROPPING ON A HIDDEN WORLD

How, specifically, do we become sensitive like this? It is at least partially about using mental filters. Many of us pay a great deal of attention to immediate gratification, and are overstimulated by the rush of information coming in from the outside world. Our brain filters this information, sorting and prioritizing it so as to make order out of chaos. The sensitivity tai chi brings us helps to refine this filter so as to focus in on the information we need from another person or from a situation. It helps us to hear, feel, and sense trends, inclinations, and information we may have spent a lifetime missing.

A few weeks ago, I saw a gardener at work in the yard next door. The owner had asked to have one of his trees removed, as it was stricken with disease and beyond saving. The gardener stood and looked for a time at the tree—a thirty-foot Madagascan Traveler's palm with a scaly trunk and a broad, flat crown—then softly touched it at a point about level with his breastbone. After a few seconds I saw the tree begin to quiver from bottom to top. The man followed the movement, adding force to it in time with the swing, swaying in effortless synchrony as the tree began to move more and more violently.

On and on the man pushed and pulled, listening to the tree's natural inclination until the trunk leaned so far over that roots began to come up out of the ground. Watching him, I was aware that I was seeing an example of listening very much like the one we cultivate in tai chi. Eventually the tree fell over, and when it did its roots came out so completely that very little digging was required to clear them.

Without tai chi we might have felt the need to be heard before we listened; practicing, we do not. To make our own noise rather than pay attention to what we can hear is to be like a doctor listening to a heart through a stethoscope while simultaneously shouting at the top of his lungs. Tai chi gently and persistently teaches us both the value and the art of listening. Having practiced for a while, a business meeting that might previously have bored or intimidated us is now a smorgasbord of information available with just a bit of sensitive listening. We can expand our ability to sense energy (qi) and intention, and to find structure not only in individual people but also in groups. We can analyze alliances and agendas without judging them, and then efficiently follow the trends we sense to best advantage.

PUSHING HANDS

The tai chi exercise most often associated with the development of sensitivity is the two-person exercise called Pushing Hands (sometimes also Sensing Hands). From a martial point of view, this is an exercise that introduces the new player to working with a partner, and provides a first step toward sparring and understanding martial combat. It is cooperative work that tests our understanding of tai chi principles such as using no force against force, relaxing, and following a partner's flow.

The ultimate goal is to contend with a partner's incoming force (a shove, a grab, a strike, a kick, the locking of a joint) by turning the dantian and waist while spiraling at the point of contact so as to effortlessly return the force from where it came. This is a useful skill both physically and emotionally, for in life outside of tai chi class we sometimes experience insults, emotional wounds, disappointments, career setbacks, blocks to our personal agenda, or other attacks or turns of fortune.

What does Pushing Hands look like? At first it is vaguely like a dance involving simple back and forward steps and the circling of arms in contact with our partner's. Sticking to each other is important, particularly later, when arm movements are mastered and steps become progressively more complicated, lower, and faster. Playing Pushing Hands we concentrate relaxation in the torso, which should feel like the light branches of the crown of a tree moving easily in the breeze. The lower half of our body is rooted into the ground, while we use our agile upper half to stick to our partner, reading what we can through the contact, always hyperaware of his movements.

Pushing Hands play reminds us that paying attention to our own personal equilibrium comes first, a message the airlines give us every time they tell us to put on our own oxygen mask first before helping others. We must lose neither our balance nor our temper. We must stay cool and calm and relaxed if we are going to be able to return a partner's force in a three-dimensional fashion that overcomes him naturally and without effort.

PUSHING HANDS AS DIPLOMATIC CURRENCY

In 2009 I traveled to China to research a novel I was writing. One Sunday morning I went to Shanghai People's Park to play Pushing Hands. I found old masters sitting on benches drinking tea and directing their respective senior students to instruct everyone else. I joined the fray and slowly worked my way up the skill ladder, in the process discovering that Shanghai-style Pushing Hands relies quite a bit on speed and tricks. By contrast, I had learned to rely on structure and principles so as to eventually be able to reach a "solution" to any Pushing Hands "problem." Inherent in this latter approach is the view that the game is not combat but an opportunity to develop sensitivity and to test one's emotional and physical equilibrium. Accordingly, I did not feel the least bit competitive with anyone there; I was just seeking to learn. Over and over again I was "beaten," and over and over again, I figured out what had been done to me and how to counter it successfully.

I grew pretty tired and hungry after five hours of the game, but when I tried to leave the park I was instead subtly pressed in the direction of a newcomer to the gathering, a tree-trunk of a monk wearing robes, a shaven head, and a stern demeanor. I had a bad feeling about being matched with him, sensing that I was hopelessly outclassed. At first the monk went easy on me, but he soon stepped up the ferocity of his maneuvers, tossing me here and there to the amusement of the onlookers.

It is a truism that ten minutes in the ring with a trained fighter is more exhausting than a half hour's swim in a cold sea. This is because in a fight, the muscles are tight with anticipation, adrenaline is flowing, and for most people relaxation is a wishful, distant concept displaced by intense focus on the here and now. As a bridge between gentle, peaceful, contemplative solo practice and the raw misery of combat, however, Pushing Hands moves us in the right direction by allowing us to cultivate our skills in a safe environment. While we may end up sitting down hard on our tailbone during a rousing match, we most certainly will not receive a killing punch or a knife to the belly.

I wanted the monk to remain interested in me, for the longer he played with me the more I learned. Even though I knew better than to plan or strategize, I managed to come up with a way to keep the game going. Whenever the monk attacked, rather than defending myself rigorously I gave in, then immediately performed on him the precise technique he had used on me. After about a dozen exchanges, he suddenly jumped back from me as if he had been shocked, threw his hands in the air, laughed loudly, and told me, in halting English, that my tai chi was not too bad. This brought a rousing round of applause from the other players for their "round eye" compatriot from the other side of the world.

It was a magical moment.

At the highest level of Pushing Hands we lose the distinction between our partner and ourselves. As the black-and-white tai chi symbol suggests, players become one complete system. As our ability to empathize grows, we lose the very notion of other, the sense of me and him. Gone are the senses of antagonism, preservation, agenda, reaction or even ego. We become skilled tai chi diplomats, or at least negotiators, and we become hyper-aware of ourselves as well. Once we have practiced to this level of achievement, we come to realize that conflict can often be effectively transcended.

SENSUALITY, SEX, AND LONGEVITY

The increased awareness and sensitivity that tai chi brings spills over into every area of our life. Improving our balance and looking for harmony in the various postures, we more readily register our own emotional shifts and cycles. We become similarly keyed into the moods and energy of those around us. While this change can make us more sensitive to negative emotions (we may, for example, gradually become less tolerant of mainstream news feeds, violent books or films, loud noises, and spicy foods) we also become more appreciative of art, music, and beauty.

In pursuit of the wuji mind and the balanced body, many tai chi players report that the practice helps them to feel happier, too. Perhaps the uptick in mood is what makes food taste better, good times more special, and meaningful work more satisfying. This deepening of experience extends to our appreciation of physical sensation, too. Bicycle rides on a crisp autumn day, the feel of a tropical ocean (or a nice warm bathtub), the scent of snow, the taste of fine wine on the tongue, the pleasure of a sinful dessert, or even the joy of a long, quiet walk in the country.

Naturally, being more open to connection and sensation also leads us to more exciting and fulfilling romantic relations as well. More and more people are turning toward natural ways to enhance their love lives, and the most natural way of all is to exercise. Everyone knows that exercise makes us feel sexier. Slimming down, getting stronger, seeing muscles grow, experiencing the flow of endorphins, and having more stamina makes us more interested in lovemaking and more desirable to others, too.

In energetic terms, tai chi builds sexual power in the same way it increases longevity—by enhancing the circulation of qi, life force, to vital areas including the sexual organs. In fact, a core goal of the practice (core is double entendre here because there may be no better routine for strengthening the body's muscular core than a rigorous tai chi class) is to increase the sexual essence, or jing. This word describes both male and female secretions. Taoist training teaches that absorbing the man's jing as essential to a woman's longevity, and absorbing the woman's jing as essential for the long life of the man.

The ancient Taoists on whose philosophy tai chi is based were adventurous, open-minded, and always engaged in pleasurable love lives. In fact, they saw the ultimate goal of all Taoist practices (indeed the ultimate goal of life) to be the balancing of the universal forces of yang and yin, which in this context means male and female. They made no distinction between pious and sacrilegious love but rather saw sex as a high pursuit, one essential to a fulfilled life and one that was required for optimal health and longevity. In fact, the longer and more frequent the lovemaking, the greater the benefit to both partners.

In texts humorously given to poetic hyperbole (the penis is the Jade Pole, the vulva is the Jade Gate, a good night of loving requires at least a thousand thrusts using positions such as Silkworm Spinning a Cocoon or Wild Horses Leaping), tai chi's progenitors emphasized intimacy, touching, emotional content, sexual technique, and satisfaction. It took the modern, "sexual revolution" to help those of us in the West see things the same way.

More, rather than seeing a "battle of the sexes," Taoists see a cyclical, ever-engaging interchange in which the emotional and physical satisfaction of both genders is of paramount importance. Alongside legendary male Taoist immortals—demigods with lots of girlfriends— were many famous female counterparts, goddesses who lived for thousands of years, all the while enjoying the favors of large numbers of virile young men. Balancing emotional and physical processes and extremes in the mind and body of the tai chi player leads to creative unpredictability, relaxation, rhythms, self-expression, going with the flow, receiving and giving, and more. Tai chi is a laboratory in which we study our own body in depth, learning new dimensions of our physical and mental being. If our sex life is feeling dull or we are feeling stuck and just can't get rolling, tai chi may be just what we need to awaken our true, powerful sexual nature.

EXPLORATIONS

As we have learned in this chapter, if we practice tai chi solely by repeating our movements, we miss the benefits of incorporating the practice into every aspect of our life. The following exercises allow us to apply our practice immediately to eating and cultivating sexual essence (jing), two areas where our sensitivity and focus can bear great fruit.

36 Chews

SPEED AND GREED MAKE OUR CULTURE MORE ABOUT THE destination than the journey. Tai chi is more about the journey than the destination, at least in part because we become progressively better informed about the meaning of things as we proceed down the path. When it comes to fully enjoying our food, the journey is eating and the destination is feeling satisfied.

Try this exercise to enhance your eating pleasure and your health. First, put your fork down between bites. Next, chew those bites 36 times (an auspicious number in tai chi) before swallowing—moving your food around in your mouth so as to engage the various taste receptors distributed around your mouth.

All this chewing reduces the work your stomach has to do, enhancing your digestion and giving the satiety center in the brain time to register that you are full, thereby helping you avoid bloat, overeating, and weight gain. As you chew, close your eyes and bring your full attention to bear on what is in your mouth. Consider the energy you get from it, the vitamins and other subtle but vital trace nutrients, and, of course, all the wonderful flavors.

Crane Walking Qigong

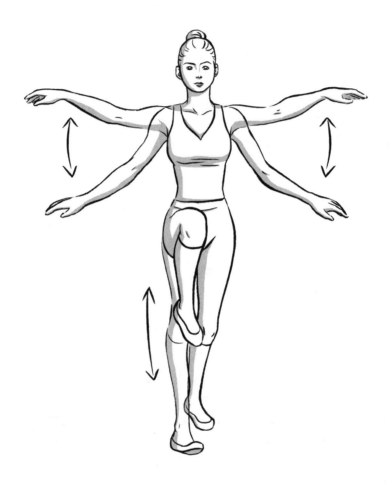

THERE ARE FIFTEEN SPECIES OF CRANES LEFT IN THE WORLD, and all are in danger of extinction. These birds symbolize longevity in China and are such powerful fliers that one type actually crests the Himalayas in its yearly migration, at times flying as high as a jetliner. Using your upper body to mimic the action of their wings in this qigong exercise loosens your shoulders and activates your lower back and kidneys, thereby building your sexual essence, or jing, which, as mentioned above, helps you to build qi.

It is best to practice the arm movements without walking first. Standing with feet shoulder-width apart, touch your thumb to the tips of your three largest fingers then lift both arms to the side, going as high as you can while still leaving your shoulders relaxed and your elbows and wrists slightly bent. Lowering your arms, keep the movement graceful and the joints soft until your arms are back at your sides and your fingers are once again in a natural position. Make sure not to hold your breath, nor to allow any tension to creep into your shoulders.

Once you are comfortable "flapping your wings" you can try combining the arm movements with some stepping. The arm and leg movements happen together. As the arms come up, the foot comes up in a large, exaggerated movement as if you are clearing an obstacle. The stepping leg bends quite a bit as it goes up and down, but the supporting leg only softens as you sink your weight into it. At the peak of the arm movements you are standing on one leg with the other tucked in, toes down, as a bird stands. Concentrate on relaxing the upper body to help you maintain your balance. As the arms go down, the foot goes down. Avoid the temptation to put down your foot too quickly. Instead, relax into your supporting leg and wait to transfer your weight onto the descending foot until it is firmly on the ground.

In the beginning it is fine to practice Crane Walking indoors, but as your skills improve you may wish to go to a park or beach and enjoy fresh air while you do this jing-building practice. Once you are comfortable with the movements, you may even wish to try it going up and down a hill, or on a mountain path. Some people enjoy listening to relaxing music through a personal player while doing this exercise, which also builds balance, leg strength, and relaxation. Remember to be as graceful and relaxed as possible as you work up to ten or fifteen minutes a day of this exercise. You will likely notice improvements in your energy and libido, too.

EXPLORATION #3

Bear Walking Qigong

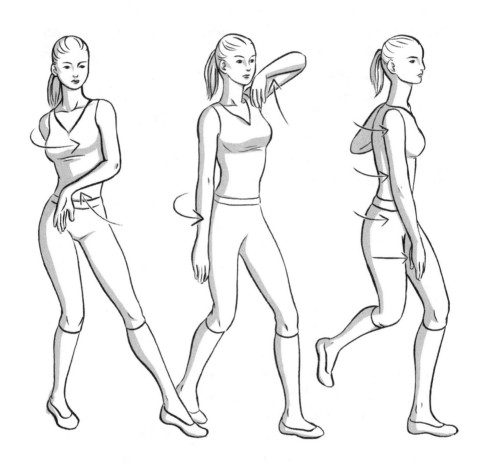

COMPARED TO CRANE WALKING, THIS QIGONG EXERCISE OFFERS a bit less benefit to leg strength and balance, but is an even more intense jing-builder. Stand with your feet together—weight evenly distributed between left and right. Begin your awareness at the top of your head and then down your body through your left side. As you do, relax and shift your weight into your left side. Feel your shoulders drop and your ribs relax as you sit down a bit into your left hip, bending your knee slightly and feeling your weight spread across the bottom of your foot. Now bring your weight back to center and try the same exercise on the right side. Repeat this any number of times, alternating sides until you are confident in the movement.

As you relax and shift your weight, you subtly allow your kidneys (and other organs) to move from side to side like a seesaw. This action stimulates circulation to the kidneys and related organs, potentiating their function and encouraging the development of jing. You can enhance this effect by incorporating your arms. Start as before, feet together and weight evenly placed left to right. Put your right hand, fingertips down, by your navel. Place your left hand close to the front of your left shoulder. Now slowly slide your right hand up your centerline while at the same time sliding your left hand behind you and down your spine to your tailbone. As one hand comes up the front, the other goes down the back.

At the end movement your hands should be in opposite positions from which they started—that is, your left hand is now by your navel and your right hand by your right shoulder. Try this movement any number of times until it flows. Now, incorporate the weight shift as before. When your right hand is coming up your centerline, shift to the right, and when your left hand is coming up shift to the left. You may even find that as you do this, your torso turns from left to right. Encourage this twist, as it further increases the stimulation of your organs.

The last element of this exercise is to try taking a step while performing the movements. As you shift into your right, take a modest step with your left. As you shift to the left and move forward, your right leg will naturally come up so that you can take a modest step on that side. Focus your awareness on the feelings of shifting, spiraling and relaxing into your supporting hip. Again, ten–fifteen minutes of this walking will both massage your kidneys and wake up your libido. Even five minutes should provide a noticeable effect.

The River of Life

There may be no physical practice anywhere more closely entwined with a system of philosophy than the martial art of tai chi is with Lao Tzu's little book, the *Tao Te Ching*. Tai chi is all about acting in accordance with Lao Tzu's idea of a universal force called the Tao, about deriving power from that Tao and using it efficiently. To get a better handle on finding the Tao in your world, consider the Tao the river of life. A river is a particularly nice metaphor, because like the Tao it pervades things, nourishes them, flows freely and powerfully, and is purely natural.

Different types of people have different relationships with this river. One kind of person walks right up to the edge and, oblivious to its presence, falls in and drowns. Another instinctively paddles across to the other bank without paying much attention to the water. A third type of person reaches the riverbank, jumps in, and swims as hard and fast as he can against the flow before becoming exhausted. A fourth kind of person jumps in with gusto and swims as hard and fast as possible *with* the current, determined to beat all other swimmers down the river.

A fifth kind of person is bent on reaching a certain goal on the opposing bank despite the bothersome distraction of the river. He calculates the speed and direction of the current and then, keeping his eye on the prize swims at just the right speed, and in precisely the right trajectory, to reach the goal. The sixth and last kind of person is the

Taoist, who simply pops into the river, turns face up and floats, enjoying every minute of the ride. When the occasional submerged rock or low-hanging branch appears, this enlightened individual simply makes a small course correction and continues his journey, all the while expending minimum effort to engage maximum sensation, satisfaction, pleasure, and efficiency.

We all know people in each of these six categories. We know folks who numb themselves to the flow of life, those who don't care about it, those whose voracious appetites drive them to an early demise, those who only care about beating others, and those who live in a world of their own creation. We know the Taoist, too, though we may not have previously recognized him as such—an individual whose personal style, grace, and inexplicable good fortune we find enviable. This is the woman who joined the company a mere four months ago and is now, impossibly, occupying the corner office. This is the man who always seems to get that dream date despite the fact that he's nothing special to look at and doesn't have much money. It's the person who always appears to be in the right place at the right time, the person everyone likes but may not especially notice, the person who seems unruffled by life's unpredictable twists and turns, the person whose life simply unfolds easily every day.

What makes a person a Taoist is the often-unconscious ability to sense the flow of life and anticipate it, to feel the speed and direction of the current in the river and then float along effortlessly. Some folks are born with this ability, but most of us acquire it through training. Tai chi, with its unique heritage, focus, flavor, and methods, is that training.

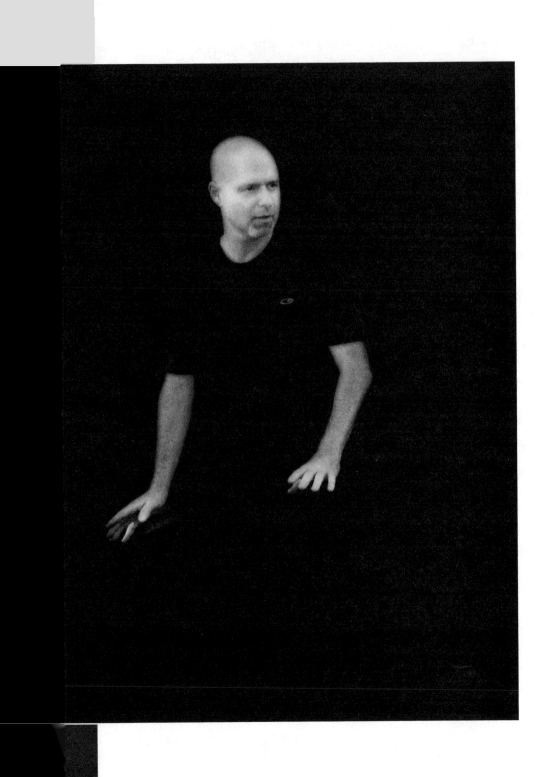

MEDICATION AND MEDITATION

During recent decades, many of us have fallen into the habit of relinquishing responsibility for our health and well-being to the commercial medical establishment. The alternative medicine revolution represents our growing desire to reclaim that responsibility. The more we can learn about the prevention and healing resources available to us, the surer we can be that we are plotting the best course to a long and healthy life. Resources that can be very useful in contending with stress and chronic conditions include mainstream biomedicine, nutritional counseling, exercise coaching, acupuncture, meditation, massage, energy work, psychological support, and mind/body practices like tai chi.

The original architects of tai chi who spent a lot of time listening to the messages of nature and turning their attention inward. Their introspection led them to insights that even modern technology cannot replace. What we can do that the ancients could not, however, is to combine our understanding of the ongoing processes of biological renewal—the way our cells continually die and are replaced, thereby remaking the very fabric of us—with information about our true nature that we gain from our tai chi practice. This synthesis allows us to elevate rejuvenation to the level of transformation and thereby change ourselves into something new and better.

Such transformation is well known in mind/body practice in general and in tai chi in particular. Kung fu action star and tai chi devotee Bruce Lee was born with one leg much shorter than the other, but his tai chi practice allowed him to transcend this challenge. My primary teacher, Master Yan, suffered from heart problems as a youngster and used his practice to heal himself when doctors said there was nothing to be done. I grew up asthmatic, overweight, and over-medicated, and used the practice to become a strong, free-breathing student of the martial arts. Whatever we believe our limitations to be, mindful practice with a meditative component and the right body mechanics can help us to transcend them. This chapter will discuss how.

MEDICATION IN MOTION

As more and more studies show that tai chi improves our balance and reduces stress, the art has become the darling of the Integrative Medicine community, and is often recommended by allopathic physicians seeking the best for their patients by employing both Eastern and Western therapeutic approaches. These healers understand the fact that most of our discomforts and ills arise from stress, and that our health depends upon our age, diet, environment, lifestyle, spiritual considerations, mental state, and genes. Ideally, that health is as resilient as bamboo and as tough as dirt, while at the same time varying within a narrow range that includes minor discomforts, the odd cold, and occasional, activity-related aches and pains.

In experiencing the ebb and flow of health, we are in the good company not only of everyday folks, but also of the most disciplined and highly trained practitioners of the various mind/body arts. Nobody can feel exactly the same way every day; what we want to avoid is big swings in our health. That's where tai chi comes in. Functioning on a variety of different levels, tai chi helps us to avoid extremes and find balance in the choices we make, the values we espouse, and the activities, causes, and goals we engage. As a physical exercise it strengthens and improves us, as a social activity it puts us in energetically uplifting company, as a martial art it helps us to stay present and aware at all times, and as a spiritual path it deepens our experience of life.

So successful is this multifaceted formula that tai chi practice can actually affect our genes. That's right. A recent study conducted at a children's hospital in Australia actually identifies genetic changes consequent to tai chi practice. and explores these changes as one explanation for tai chi's wide-ranging benefits.[1] Imagine that! Our tai chi practice can actually change what we once thought was written in stone. The result of this change is that we become different people mentally, emotionally, and physically.

More stable, clearer, quieter, and stronger, we are less likely to be plagued by a wide range of illnesses and afflictions. Worldwide scientific interest is constantly growing. At the time of this writing, the U.S. National Library of Medicine/National Institutes of Health alone lists 445 studies of the art's benefits. Here are a few highlights:

- Tai chi practice enhances the effects of immunization against shingles (herpes) by providing a measurable strengthening of the immune system.[2]
- Tai chi reduces urinary tract symptoms (and improves quality of life) in elderly patients.[3]
- Tai chi reduces the risk of bone fractures in post-menopausal women.[4]
- Tai chi reduces falls in elderly patients.[5]
- Tai chi helps rehabilitation from heart failure.[6]
- Tai chi reduces low back pain and related disability.[7]

- Tai chi reduces cellular inflammation.[8]
- Tai chi may prevent or even reverse the progression of coronary artery disease.[9]
- Tai chi improves lung function and slows down the progress of Chronic Obstructive Pulmonary Disease.[10]
- Tai chi helps osteoarthritis, rheumatoid arthritis, and fibromyalgia.[11]
- Tai chi repairs our DNA.[12] [13]
- Tai chi improves the quality of our sleep.[14]
- Tai chi reduces blood pressure.[15]
- Tai chi benefits diabetes patients.[16]
- Tai chi improves asthma in children.[17]
- Tai chi reduces tension headaches.[18]
- Tai chi facilitates recovery from severe head injury.[19]
- Tai chi helps older people retain their cardiovascular fitness.[20]
- Tai chi is great for spinal integrity.[21]
- Tai chi alleviates depression.[22]

The takeaway from reading these studies is that tai chi's health benefits are so numerous that we could be excused for thinking of the art as some kind of medical miracle. Why might this be so? Certainly we can say that tai chi benefits the circulatory system. This may be because physical relaxation, particularly of the extremities, results in a relaxation of the muscular walls of the peripheral arteries and capillary bed, thereby reducing back pressure on the heart and allowing it to contract without strain. Relaxation of the muscles through which veins pass may, in turn, allows easier venous drainage of deoxygenated blood back into the heart, thereby also reducing the pumping burden. These phenomena may tone the heart muscle while stabilizing blood pressure either up or down, as needed. As noted earlier, tai chi's spiraling, twisting action moves blood and lymph in much the way we wring water from a towel. Tai chi's effects on the nervous system are at least as complex. An example is tai chi's effect on proprioception (knowing where you are in your physical environment). Proprioceptive competence diminishes with age, but whereas this decline was previously ascribed to the death of sensory neurons, it is now known to be degradation in the relationship between sensory input and attention. In other words, our brain and our feet forget how to talk to each other, and tai chi helps them to remember. This revival contributes greatly to balance and thence to avoiding the sort of morbid falls—a great preoccupation for all of us as we age—that often spell hospitalization and the beginning of a downward spiral from which we may never recover.

The fact that tai chi stimulates new neural growth, even in the brain, may explain how it benefits the immune system, depression, and ADHD. There is some speculation that tai chi, like acupuncture, may move qi through the layered matrix of what we call the fascia, or connective tissue. In an amazing turn of scientific inquiry stimulated by the growing interest in tai chi in general and qi in particular, it may turn out that there is an entire communications network in the body that Western science has yet to recognize, a web through which electrical impulses and chemical messengers travel, conveying information to and from the brain and between organ systems. If so, tai chi may directly influence the intimate interchange between mind and meat. Whatever the exact mechanism, tai chi certainly improves physical fitness by improving flexibility and strengthening both joints and the muscular core. As such it is a prescription for longevity and vitality, a strong defensive tool against aging and decrepitude.

LIVING SLOWER, LONGER, AND BETTER

Imagine that we are in our last few moments of life, having just stepped off the curb and been hit by a bus. As we lie on the street with our life slipping away, we hear people screaming and we see someone dialing 911. We hear the wail of an approaching ambulance and realize, in a place beyond pain and terror, that it will arrive too late. Surely we don't want our last thought to be, "That was fast, but at least I got a lot done." Instead, we all hope that when our time comes, we have a feeling of satisfaction, a sense that we have fully engaged the people in our lives, that we tried the things we wanted to try, that we made a contribution to the world, that we leave content with having been present for each and every moment, and that our dreams, if not fully realized, have at least been avidly and joyously pursued.

Living this way means slowing down and paying attention, and the moment we make an effort to do that, we become aware of just how addicted we are to being titillated, distracted, and entertained. A little yin/yang war ensues in which we alternately crave constant stimulation on one hand and peaceful tranquility on the other. At any given moment on any given day one or the other side will win, but one way we can begin to tilt the balance in favor of relaxation and focus is to practice tai chi. Because the art requires focus and involves movement, it results in natural mindfulness and organic slowness. Pushed and pulled along too quickly and in too many directions, we feel stressed and respond with illness; slow and mindful we are able to prioritize what needs to be done, discard what doesn't, and even enjoy the doing.

Until very recently, a great premium was placed on multitasking. Conventional wisdom had it that a brain able to multitask is a brain competently engaged in meeting the demands of today's busy lifestyle. The latest information, however, suggests what mindfulness practitioners have known all along, namely that doing too many things at the same time actually causes a "brown-out" of the brain. What we are choosing when we divide our brainpower this way is to do many things at once, and all of them poorly. It turns out that we are much better off focusing purely on one task at a time, be it surfing the Web, driving, texting, wiping up a toddler's spill, cleaning the house, penning a business plan, working on an annual report, or doing our expense account. Talking to our boss on a conference call while touching up our makeup and checking our e-mail messages is a sure way to miss something important or say something we will regret.

Certainly we all need to act quickly at times; our very survival may depend upon it. Sometimes, too, we may need to handle multiple inputs. Yet multitasking is not something we naturally choose to do; in modern living it is most often a response to being forced to get a certain number of things done within a specified time frame. A well-considered life does not always mean rebelling or ignoring the rules, but many people who accomplish truly meaningful things will not allow themselves to be rushed. Deliberate, mindful, and focused, they are free of frivolous demands, compulsions, and projects. Not addicted to a pace of life set by outside forces whose motivations are almost always driven by their own profit or interests, this kind of person, the sage we all can be if we choose, concentrates his or her energy effectively on those tasks that really matter. As proof of such concentration, one study shows that tai chi even improves our math computation skills![23]

It is not only our external performance that suffers when mindfulness fails, but also our internal environment. Doing too much at the same time is a great stressor. Our brain interprets a drumming rainstorm of input as an existential crisis (a tiger is in the village, the local warlord is invading, the cave is flooding) and responds with a rush of stress hormones. These hormones help us to do what we need to do right then and there, but if we live with them day in and day out our health suffers. Tai chi enables us to break this bad habit and preserve our health.

Imagine if we all lived this way. Imagine if we were willing to stop grasping at things we don't need, rushing around chasing measures that don't matter, keeping up a pace so frenetic we never figure things out. Taking time to notice the marvels of everyday life sounds so simple, so utopian, so hopelessly out of touch with real life…but what is actually real? The world is as we make it, and we can make it different. Imagine the global shift we would see if everyone slowed down enough to notice what's really going on.

WHY MEDITATION

For the first nine months after conception, the whoosh and rumble of our mother's breath defines our world and is the metronome by which we sing the song of life. Small wonder, then, that in later years our own breath becomes a gateway to a most effective antidote to the stress of modern living, a bomb shelter from the weapons of mass distraction our culture wields, a refuge wherein we can rediscover the basic ingredients of what it means to be alive. That refuge is called meditation, and it provides the silence between the notes of life without which there would be no melody.

As it is for physical tai chi practice, the scientific literature on the benefits of meditation is growing daily. In fact, the number of studies that pertain to meditation listed by the U.S. National Library of Medicine/National Institutes of Health is nearly three times larger than it is for tai chi. Highlights include:

- Meditation relieves anxiety.[24] [25]
- Meditation is a potential therapy for autism.[26]
- Meditation prevents acute respiratory infections.[27]
- Meditation benefits profound depression and eating disorders.[28]
- Meditation benefits irritable bowel syndrome.[29]
- Meditation is useful in controlling blood pressure.[30] [31]
- Meditation reduces work stress.[32]
- Meditation helps schizophrenia.[33]
- Meditation helps fibromyalgia.[34]
- Meditation helps multiple sclerosis.[35]
- Meditation may reduce the need for sleep.[36]
- Like tai chi, meditation may positively affect our DNA (shorten telomeres).[37]
- Meditation helps tinnitus (ringing in the ears).[38]
- Meditation helps patients with cancer.[39] [40] [41]
- Meditation may positively affect our rate of aging.[42]

While filming my own documentary on meditation, I interviewed researchers at Harvard and other august institutions who showed me that meditation actually changes the structure of our brain to reverse the loss of brain tissue normally seen with aging.[43]

Clearly, there is something to the way meditation affects our physical structure, our immune system, and the way our body balances inputs and responds with stress hormones and physiological changes. Meditation may be right for us if we:

- Would like to make the good times last longer.
- Would like to find value in both challenges and chores.
- Prefer books to television because we can lose ourselves more fully when we bring our imagination to bear actively rather than passively.
- Would like our lovemaking to last longer and feel better.
- Desire more intensity and focus to all areas of life.
- Like the idea of carrying around an always-accessible personal refuge from the maelstrom of the world.
- Are constantly aware that in speeding up our lives we are merely racing to our inevitable end.

Meditation practice may have a variety of goals. These days it seems most often used to combat stress, but it may also be employed to heal, to relax, to increase specific abilities, or to probe the mysteries of the universe with the most significant tool at our disposal—our mind. It may be performed in a solitary place or in a group, and it may be conducted in silence, to music, or following the spoken word down a path of guided visualization. It is capable of providing spiritual insights and even thrills, and of calming mood swings and emotional suffering. It may be done standing up, sitting down, lying prone, floating in a sensory deprivation tank, while riding a motorcycle (yes, it is possible to become meditative at speed) or, of course, while doing tai chi. What meditation requires most is mindfulness, the art of being totally and completely attentive to the present moment.

We learned a great deal about meditation at the turn of the last century, when Nobel Prize laureate Dr. Wilder Penfield attempted to "map" the connections between parts of the body and specific areas of the brain. He wanted to discover, for example, what part of the brain controls our hands, what part controls our feet, where in the brain we experience sadness or euphoria, and more. To produce his map, Penfield needed his brains alive and his subjects awake and talking. Fortunately, while the skull has sensory nerves in it, the brain does not, so Penfield could numb the skull and go ahead and poke around in the brain without causing pain. Mapping, it turned out, was a process of stimulating with electrodes, then asking the patient what he or she was experiencing, and noting the answers.

Those answers gave Penfield his map, but they also gave him a wonderfully exciting mystery. Rather than simply saying, "Yum, mustard," when Penfield stimulated his brain, the patient was able to say, "When you use the first needle, I taste salt, but when you use the second I taste mustard on my tongue." The way the patient communicated suggested that there were, in fact, two people, the one who was speaking and the one that voice referred to as "I." Penfield realized that in order to phrase things that way, the patient had to be both able to directly experience the needle and to be aware of the experiment from some place deep within, or high above.

There's more. When Penfield stimulated a place in the brain that made the patient clench his fist, he used such language as, "Look, I'm going to do that again, this time try to resist the clenching." Guess what happened? The fist didn't clench so tight! Again this suggested that the person whose hand was moving and the person who was trying to stop the hand from moving were not one and the same! Penfield called the person he was talking to the "watcher."

In Taoist meditation—and indeed in other metaphysical traditions as well—the phenomenon of the watcher is well known. Some systems of inner development go so far as to name a particular watcher as the "real" consciousness inside us. It might be the fifth one, for example: the I watching the I watching the I watching the I watching the I. Trying to find the watcher within us can be a very interesting experience. If we spend a little time at it we discover that we can go "up a few levels" without any special training at all. The best way to do it is simply to sit quietly, eyes closed, in a peaceful place, and pay attention. The first watcher (the second I) will immediately appear and we will be able to see ourself in our mind's eye, sitting quietly. Next, we can try to see the I that just saw the I sitting quietly. If we can manage that—not typical for someone without meditation training but certainly possible—then we keep going until we can add no further watchers.

Simply recognizing the fact of multiple levels of consciousness (or multiple identities) within a single mind provides an instantly useful tool, especially when we are stressed, fearful, or angry. There are multiple emotional states within us at all times, and with a little practice we can scale the ladder of watchers until we find one who is cool, calm, collected, not angry or stressed, not in the throes of passion or despair, but one who has perspective, the watcher who is the highest, best, truest expression of ourself.

BRINGING ENERGY AND MIND TOGETHER

The more experienced we become at tai chi practice, the more meditative our movements become. Indeed, over time the distinction between specifically meditative techniques in tai chi and form practice (as well as the repetitive performance of single movements—so-called "solo exercises") blurs. Contrary to popular opinion, meditation is not doing nothing; rather it is an active process that may have a wide variety of goals and purposes in the context of different arts, belief systems, and traditions. As part of a tai chi program, meditation helps us to build a balanced, harmonious, wuji mind. This is important because when we are distracted, anxious, irritable, or depressed we cannot be completely present for our physical training and thus, by definition, are not practicing tai chi. Not only does meditation quiet our wandering mind and reduce our emotional volatility, it also makes us more sensitive and aware—two qualities highly prized in our art.

Spiritually, as tai chi meditators we are gradually lifted from a constrained, ego-centered existence into awareness of our integral place in a fabric that includes everything in the universe. Experienced as a moving meditation, tai chi becomes more rooted and relaxed. Paradoxically, paying great attention to slow movements and the sensations they offer improves our ability to move quickly when circumstances require. Our forms become smoother and more intricate as our mind brings awareness and emotional content to our movements. At some point in our practice, we come to feel that we are completely clear and calm—that something other than our muscles is moving us through our patterns. This something is qi, and as we experience its presence and flow, it is natural to want more of it.

While physical tai chi practice refines and redistributes the qi, according to Taoist tradition there is only one way to actually increase the quantity of qi we possess, and that is to meditate, a process that both connects us to the world around us (to heaven above us and earth below, in the Taoist view) and encourages the energy that comes from that connection to pervade every nook and cranny of the body, vitalizing our organs, muscle, and bone while growing the mind toward enlightenment.

Broadly put, the energy coming in from Bai Hui (the Crown Point) and through the paired Yong Quan (Bubbling Spring) points at the bottom of the foot circulates along two related paths the Taoists call the "Heavenly Circles." (See Chapter 5.) At the first level of our tai chi development it moves through the Lesser Heavenly Circle, which is confined to the torso, and eventually it moves through the Larger Heavenly Circle, which encompasses the entire body.

Consider these circles thin, pure, cool streams generated by the nature of the human body in its dance with heaven and earth rather than physical pathways or roads. They cannot be smelled or heard or tasted or felt from the outside. They flow whether or not we are aware of them, but are most enhanced, both in interior dynamics and external connection, when we achieve that specific melding of a properly aligned body and a relaxed, open mind we call wuji. Thus mentally and physically relaxed, our energy circles open. The more those circles open, the more qi flows within us. Increased qi grows our spirit, increasing our awareness of reality and connects us to the Tao.

EXPLORATIONS

There are many different techniques that fall under the umbrella of tai chi meditation. As we have already seen, we can use solo exercises, form practice, and even partner play to achieve meditative results while relaxing, spiraling, and rooting. The following explorations, however, are about meditating in physical stillness. Each one offers a different combination of supportive, comfortable posture, and directed mental focus. The result is a good range of meditation exercises. Use any or all of them to cultivate the habit of meditating every day. Try not to skip a day, even if you can only find time to meditate for a few minutes. Extend the period of your meditation whenever you are able. There is no upward limit. The more you meditate, the stronger the physical, mental, emotional, and energetic results will be.

Reclining with the Breath

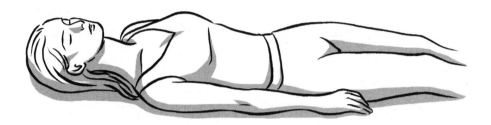

MEDITATING WHILE LYING DOWN IS A GOOD CHOICE WHEN YOU
are very tired or recuperating from an illness or injury. Choose a quiet
place where you will not be disturbed. If quiet is hard to find, you
may wish to use some good foam earplugs or a music player with
headphones. Choose music that does not compel you with words or a
melody, but which provides an auditory curtain for any noise you cannot avoid. There are many good choices for meditation music, ranging from Asian and New Age selections to Native American flute
tracks, and even gentle electronica.

It is best to lie on a hard surface, or at least a firm one, so that your
spine is straight, your back flat, and your chest open. Using a yoga mat
or towel over a tile floor or short-pile carpet offers a fine meditation
platform. Avoid a soft bed or couch, as when you sink into a yielding
surface your weight is unevenly distributed and certain muscles may
have trouble relaxing. More, if you are too comfortable you may fall
asleep.

Place your hands palms up by your sides, or lightly folded across
your belly, just below your navel, in the region of your Dantian. If you
do fold your hands, place them palms down and one on top of the
other so that the Laogong (pericardium 8) acupuncture points in the
center of each palm line up. Your feet should be uncrossed, toes up or

slightly splayed, and your face should be uncovered so as not to obstruct your breathing in any way.

Position your tongue so that the tip falls comfortably against the roof of the mouth, behind the front teeth. The exact position of the tip of the tongue is a complex subject in Taoist meditation, as it affects the energetic flow of the body. Interestingly, your body will instinctively know where your tongue tip should touch, so don't overthink the subject. Just be sure there is no tension in your mouth as you leave it comfortably closed and inhale and exhale through your nose.

In the beginning, it is useful to keep track of the time you spend meditating. Use a kitchen timer, cell phone timer, or watch to do this. Start with five or ten minutes and work up to half an hour. See if you can stay present and awake, but if you can't, don't worry. It simply means you are tired. Rest. The tai chi way is the natural way, and especially in meditation you don't want to force anything.

Once you are ready to begin, close your eyes and shift your attention to your breathing. Notice that the mere act of watching your breath may cause you to hold it, or result in rapid or strained breathing. Let that state pass as you sink comfortably into the surface beneath you. Concentrate on your breath as a way of keeping your mind focused. It can be very helpful to count your breath as you lie there, with each inhale and exhale cycle comprising one whole breath. Note the quality of your breath (thin, full, forced, slow, fast) and look for catches or snags in your inhale and exhale. See if you can't smooth the process.

Once you are finished with your session, divide the number of breaths you took by the number of minutes you meditated. The resulting number is your breaths per minute. Over time, you should try to get this number to be as low as possible, as it is a sign of your level of relaxation. Less than tens breaths a minute is quite good, less than five is a sign you are very relaxed. Once you have recovered from your illness or injury, or once you have simply gained the ability to stay focused on your breath, and feel ready for another exercise, proceed to the next exploration.

Sitting with the
Lesser Heavenly Circle

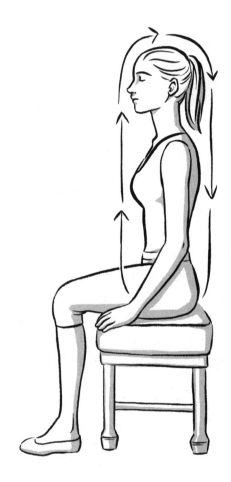

IN THIS EXERCISE WE WILL COMBINE A SITTING MEDITATION
posture with training awareness of the Lesser Heavenly Circle described above. Sitting meditation is useful on days when we are too
tired to stand, or have worked our legs very hard in training. It can

also be a good choice for short sessions in public places like airports or on buses or trains, as we can do it stealthily, without anyone around us realizing we are practicing.

To begin, find a straight-back chair and slide your rear end all the way up against it to help you keep your spine erect. Keep your feet flat on the ground and your knees at the width of your hips. Fold your hands over the navel as in lying meditation or place them on the knees either palm up or palm down. Your shoulders should be down and relaxed and your head should feel lifted by a string leading from heaven to Bai Hui (the Crown Point). As in the previous exploration, allow the tip of your tongue to find a comfortable resting place behind your upper front teeth. Feel free, once again, to use either earplugs or music to insulate you from distracting sounds.

Spend a few initial minutes with your eyes closed, watching your thoughts. Don't strive to empty your mind or stop thinking, as your so-called "monkey mind"—that lively, chattering companion that lives inside your head—is a necessary function of being alive. As thoughts arise, let them go. New ones will come. Watch them as you become more aware and sensitive to the feelings, tempos, and cycles within your body, everything from twitches and itches to transient aches or sensations of temperature.

After a few quiet minutes of just being present, turn your attention to your Dantian, the place behind and just below your navel. Imagine a teapot sitting there, with the spout aiming backward toward your spine. The pot is full of a blue tea that begins to bubble as you apply the heat of your body to it. Get a clear mental image of the bubbling pot, and as the tea boils, visualize a blue mist leaving the spout. See the mist float up and back. Once it touches your spine, see it rise from vertebra to vertebra, climbing upward in a blue line toward the base of your skull.

The blue line follows the centerline of your head up to Bai Hui at your crown, then traces its way down the center of your forehead. Next, it follows the line of your nose down to your upper lip, where it turns inward to greet the tip of your tongue. From there, the blue line goes down your tongue and into your throat. At the hollow of your throat it joins the centerline of the front of your body and goes down your chest all the way to just below your navel, where it heads inward to refill the teapot and be warmed again for another circuit of your body.

Spend some time visualizing this circuit. Again using a timer of your choice, start with a five-minute session and then add a minute a day, gradually increasing your ability to visualize the blue line. Keep at it until you are doing the work for thirty or forty minutes each day. After a few weeks of sessions you may start to feel the effects of the energy moving through your body along this important route. Every one of us has a different experience with meditation and unique results, too. You may experience relief from any chronic pain, a lessening of anxiety, an increase in your daily energy, a resistance to negative or off-balancing emotions, a new clarity and focus in your thinking, and improved concentration. Once you have spent some time with this exercise, you are ready for the next one.

Standing with the Greater Heavenly Circle

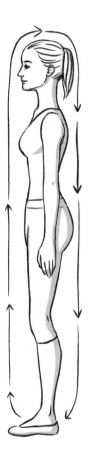

THE HOLY GRAIL OF TAI CHI MEDITATION IS CALLED ZHAN ZHUANG or "standing pole" training, and requires an upright stance. Meditating while standing upright might seem counterintuitive to us Westerners, but there are good reasons for doing it. Primary among these is that the posture described here—the classic wuji position—opens all our meridians and allows our qi to flow freely, leading to the most powerful meditative results in all of Taoist practice.

According to Traditional Chinese Medicine, the very best time of day to do standing meditation is between 11 p.m. and 2 a.m. This may not be a practical time, although if you go to bed early, rise to stand for a while, and then return to sleep you can derive great benefit. Earlier in the evening is the next best choice, followed by standing in the afternoon. Standing in meditation in the morning may yield the least benefit, but is still far better than not standing in meditation at all.

To begin, find a comfortable, safe, quiet place. This particular form of meditation is best done outdoors in nice weather, in a park, near a pond or lake or even on the beach, so long as you are not exposed to wind. If you can't find a suitable outdoor location, find an indoor space that has good ventilation, perhaps some plants, and offers an environment in which you can relax. Wear loose, comfortable clothing and flat shoes—no heels—that are thin enough for you to feel the ground through them. Place your feet parallel to each other and shoulder-width apart. As in previous explorations, place the tip of your tongue on the roof of your mouth behind your front teeth. Once again, you may use earplugs or a music player to insulate you from unwanted noise, and again, too, you will want to use some kind of watch or timer to keep track of the duration of your practice session.

Adjust your stance so that there is no pain in your knees, ankles, or any other joints. See if you can release the tension in your hips, allowing them to settle in such a way that your thighs rotate slightly inward. Once again your head should feel as if it is suspended from heaven and you should feel very rooted and planted in your feet. Drop your lower back so that you "fill" the acupuncture point Ming Men (Heaven's Gate) opposite your navel. Doing so flattens the natural, inward spinal curve and takes some pressure off your back. Fold your hands over your Dantian as you did in the previous exercises.

Now, spend some time letting your breath settle down. Watch your thoughts and adjust your stance so that you feel comfortable. Relax sequentially downward in your pose, starting at the top of your head and continuing through the chest, abdomen, hips, legs, and all the way to your feet. Your breath should not be forced, and it doesn't matter whether you belly breathe (inhale the belly swells, exhale the belly contracts) or reverse breathe (inhale the belly contracts, exhaling the belly swells) so long as you watch for snags and glitches, and smooth the breath as best you can.

As you stand, you will feel pressure in your thigh muscles. That is natural and desirable, as one of the benefits of this meditation posture is that it strengthens your legs. If and when the muscle burn is too much, come up in your stance a bit to relieve it. While it can be helpful to sink deeply and bend the knees and hips ever more as you grow stronger, if you become too uncomfortable it is better to "shake out" your arms and legs and then resume meditating than it is to endure pain. Trying to tough it out will only mean that you are thinking of nothing but your discomfort, a topic not particularly helpful when it comes to relaxing and developing a clear mind.

Once your breathing is quiet, it is time to imagine the Greater Heavenly Circle. Begin by closing your eyes and applying your attention on the Bubbling Well points at the center of the ball of each foot. Imagine that you can feel the energy coming into your foot right up out of the ground in the same blue line you used in the sitting exercise. Imagine that the blue line goes back to your heel and then to your ankle and rises up the back of your calf. As you relax ever more deeply into your stance, imagine that the downward pressure of your weight is creating a pump to your qi, raising it ever higher up the back of both legs until the two blue lines come together at your tailbone. As you continue to breathe, relax, and sink more deeply into the ground, imagine the blue line of qi rising up your spine to the base of your neck. Again, as it did in the previous exercise, see it go over the top of your head, down your nose, into your mouth, across your tongue, down your throat, down the centerline of your body all the way to your Dantian, where you previously located the teapot.

This time, however, instead of seeing the qi collect in the pot, imagine that it enters the teapot but continues flowing down the inside of both legs all the way back to the Bubbling Well points and thence back to the ground. Rather than concentrating on heating and distributing the qi in this particular visualization exercise, you want to imagine the fullness of the circuit. See if you can feel the qi circulate. Remember that the force of your relaxation is the pump that drives the circuit. The more you relax, the more powerfully the qi moves through you.

Start with a few minutes of standing and use your timing device and discipline to add a minute a day every day for a month. Along the way to half an hour a day you will experience some muscle soreness and even some stiffness too. Don't worry. This will ease as you get stronger. If standing becomes uncomfortable for you, or if there is a particular day when your mind is just too cluttered or disturbed to stand, you can skip a day, although standing is a great recipe for the disquieted mind and it is always worth trying, if only for a few minutes.

Even though it may be difficult at first, standing meditation is the single most important exercise in your tai chi arsenal, and one you will come to value and enjoy greatly over time. As you get the hang of it, be kind to yourself and suspend judgment of your progress. There is no rush. Emphasize the journey, not the destination, and you will feel the results in a matter of weeks, if not days.

What might those results be? First and foremost you can expect to build a foundation for the rest of your tai chi practice, a strong set of legs and a keen ability to relax and sink inside the sort of alignment the art demands. Second, you can expect an increase in your overall level of vitality, strength, and energy. Third, you can expect better concentration, more restful sleep, and increased emotional equanimity. Last, but not least, you may experience a deepening sense of quiet in your life, one that leads to greater insight, sensitivity, and compassion.

Acupuncture Points for Tai Chi Meditation and Practice

RELAXATION FROM THE TOP DOWN IS AN ESSENTIAL ELEMENT OF both moving tai chi practice and tai chi meditation. Knowing the acupuncture points to focus on at each level of the body helps us to visualize this process more precisely, and because qi follows yi (energy follows intention) this knowledge augments tai chi's health benefits.

The points important in tai chi practice include: Bai Hui (Governing Vessel 20, Crown Point): Located at the crown of the head, at the center (back to front) of the midline (left to right). This is the point from which we imagine ourselves to be suspended during practice, lending lightness, agility, and a straight spine.

Jian Jing (Gall Bladder Meridian 21, Shoulder Well): Located at the apex of the front of the shoulder, in the hollow at the top, in line with the nipple. Considering this point helps to release tension in the shoulder and assures that it is down and relaxed.

Zhong Fu (Lung Meridian 1, Middle Mansion): This is the soft area just medial to the shoulder, near the front of the armpit. Softening it makes sure that the chest muscles are relaxed, though it is important not to hunch over or close the chest when relaxing it.

Qi Men (Liver Meridian 14, Cycle Gate): This point is just below the nipple on each side. Softening it helps to smooth breathing and release tension in the chest, easing pressure on the heart.

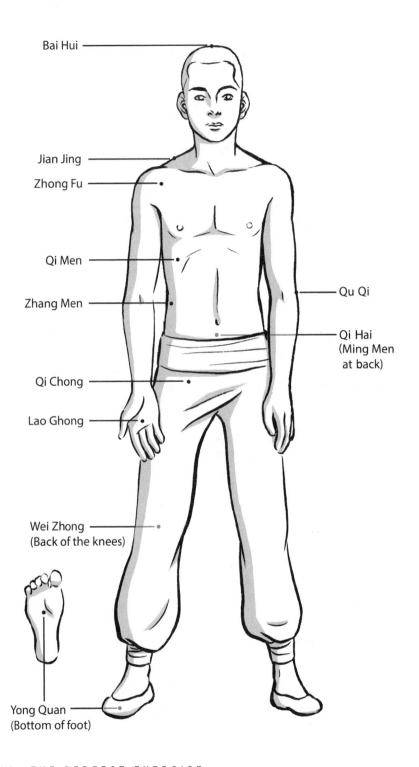

Bai Hui

Jian Jing

Zhong Fu

Qi Men

Zhang Men

Qi Chong

Lao Ghong

Wei Zhong
(Back of the knees)

Yong Quan
(Bottom of foot)

Qu Qi

Qi Hai
(Ming Men
at back)

Zhang Men (Liver Meridian 13, Bright Door): Near the floating rib, approximately two inches above the navel and six inches from the midline. Breathing into the belly helps to soften this point.

Qi Chong (Stomach Meridian 30, Surging Qi): Between the navel and the inguinal crease but closer to the latter. This point softens when we sit back and down into the hips as if taking a seat on a high stool, indicating correct alignment of the pelvic area. Relaxing it straightens the lower back, flattening the curve there and filling Ming Men.

Ming Men (Governing Vessel 4, Life Gate): Perhaps the single most important point in tai chi, it is on the lower back, directly opposite the navel. It is essential that this area feels inflated, not concave during practice, which helps in correct pelvic orientation, free breathing, and relaxation of the torso.

Qi Hai (Conception Vessel 6, Sea of Qi): One and a half finger-widths below the navel, this point demarcates the area around which the Dantian rotates. Settling into this area assists us in relaxing and achieving correct alignment.

Feng Shi (Gall Bladder Meridian 31, Wind Market): This point is where the tip of the middle finger lands on the side of our thigh when we are standing with our arms at our sides during tai chi meditation. Keeping the finger there, and aware, when we are standing helps leg strength and low back pain.

Wei Zhong (Bladder Meridian 40, Popliteal Center): At the center of the back of the knee, softening this point while in standing meditation helps us to keep the right amount of tension in the leg and the right arch to the knee, neither bent too much nor locked.

Yong Quan (Kidney Meridian 1, Bubbling Spring): On the sole of the foot just behind the middle of the ball, this is the point at which we center our weight while standing and doing the tai chi form.

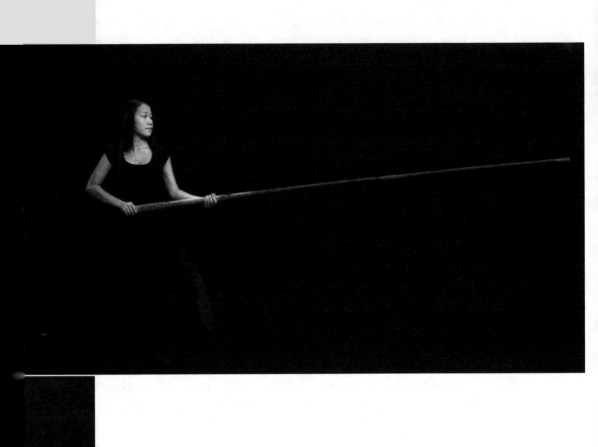

> "With the fruits of victory desist;
> Never seek to break a beaten foe,
> And flaunt no prowess with the victory,
> Assert no strength, show no pride;
> Be a victor against your will,
> A victor who will not dominate."
>
> TAO TE CHING, V. 30 (MOSS ROBERTS, TRANSLATOR)

TAI CHI KUNG FU

In martial arts terms and in martial arts circles, tai chi is inaccurately seen at best as a pasture for hard-core has-beens and at worst the sole terrain of elderly people who wish to recover from a heart attack, move without arthritis pain, or commune with butterflies and nature. It was not always so. One hundred and fifty years ago, tai chi (ch'uan) was seen as the most exalted branch of Chinese boxing—a system that was taught to imperial bodyguards who had access to the best fighting systems in the land. More recently than that, many tai chi masters built their reputations on their scrapping skills. Indeed, some still do.

MARTIAL TAI CHI IN THE MODERN WORLD

While even today there are players genuinely entranced by tai chi's martial dimension, many seem to want to stick their fingers in their ears about the subject, lumping traditional martial training together with the kind of random violence that increasingly seems to lead to tragedy in our world. I can certainly understand this. Indeed those first to embrace tai chi on our shores were peace-and-love movement hippies who, in the 1960s and early 1970s, read the seminal Taoist works of Alan Watts and studied with early American tai chi masters such as Marshall Ho'o in Los Angeles and Cheng Manqing in New York.

Despite those early American associations, tai chi is and always will be a martial art. If it evolves to lose its martial dimension, it may be something valuable and new, but it will not be tai chi. Without understanding and embracing the martial side of the practice, one not only denies tai chi's heritage but ironically loses its healing and revitalizing power. Tai chi is so empowering precisely because it is designed to move energy and to contend with force. We must celebrate tai chi's original intent, for it is that very practicality that makes the art so immediately testable, and in this way so different from other mind/body practices.

Unlike street fighting and hand-to-hand combat for policemen and soldiers in kill-or-be-killed situations, traditional martial arts training—in tai chi or any other discipline—builds character, discipline, focus, perseverance, compassion, humility, a sense of service, and a spiritual link to a larger world. The fact that as we get older and wiser our opponents become both thugs and the degenerative diseases of aging does not mean we should turn away from tai chi's martial core. In fact, if we are not martially competent—at least within the context of the average tai chi school—then something is amiss in our understanding and application of philosophy and principles. What we do with our martial competence is another matter. I am in no way advocating a confrontational attitude or a combative life. Rather, I am saying that the very same movements that work in contending with a physical attack are the ones that best help us relax and bolster our health.

Tai chi power is a path to peace and harmony, not only because of body mechanics and energetics, but because of the art's social dimensions. We can and must cultivate ourselves with tai chi, but in the end developing a tai chi community is essential if we want to apply our physical skills. Energetically and logistically, you must have people around you—and cooperative people at that—if you are going to successfully learn the art. Doesn't sound very aggressive and antisocial, does it?

IMPORTANT MARTIAL CONCEPTS

A deep understanding of tai chi requires that we view the art through a battlefield lens. Why the word battlefield? Because tai chi is an art designed for the theater of war. The system the Li and Chen families conspired to create (see Watercourse — Rooted in a Wondrous Past) was not intended as a health practice, nor even to save the skin of upper class gentlemen abroad in the city; it was, in fact, a secret, closely guarded art intended for bodyguards, private mercenaries, and soldiers. Being a battlefield art meant that it relied a great deal upon weapons, and that kicks and punches—ineffective against mounted opponents or those wearing heavy armor—were eschewed in favor of throws, pushes, and locks. This is important, because although there are brutal strikes in tai chi, they are neither primary nor exclusively characteristic of the art.

Momentum is important on the battlefield. Attacks occur with speed and ferocity, carrying with them the weight of both battle gear and mortal intent. Tai chi's founding fathers treated such assaults for the forces of nature they were, and looked both to Lao Tzu's *Tao Te Ching* and to the classical *I Ching* for guidance in understanding such forces (remember, philosophy is one of the three legs of the tripod upon which tai chi is built). As a result, tai chi specializes in the efficient redirection of force. Interestingly, despite the battlefield origins of the art and the sometimes-spectacular manifestations of its techniques, the tai chi response is always proportional to the attack. This is because we borrow an opponent's energy to fuel what we do. Our strikes frequently feature explosive shaking or vibrating energy known as fajing. In addition tai chi has a very complex system of joint locking, or qinna.

To understand better how tai chi borrows energy, consider the tai chi fighter as you would the transmission in a car. Like the transmission, we want all our gears to be well oiled and spinning freely. Like the transmission we rely completely on the engine of our opponent's moves. Like the transmission, we depend upon our structure and design to accomplish our mission. Unlike the transmission, which conducts force to the ground through the wheels, tai chi movements conduct force to a wide range of places but ultimately always back to the opponent who issued them. More, as tai chi players are not rigid machines functioning only along two-dimensional planes but organic, three-dimensional, conscious entities capable of expressing a wide range of intentions, we also have many possible options regarding how, where, in what direction, and at what angle we can use the incoming force.

One thing a properly functioning transmission does not do is to resist the force of the engine. Similarly, the tai chi player never pits force against force. This is a central tenet of Lao Tzu's brand of Taoism, which exhorts us always to be like water. Water rounds peaks, carves valleys, and tames mountains on its way to low places, forever avoiding conflict. So, too, is it with the tai chi combatant, who flows around an opponent's force even if her own is superior, who drains none of her own qi in grunting contests, who handles power elegantly, sparingly, three-dimensionally, and above all efficiently. If anything feels effortful, we have misunderstood tai chi.

Battling like water requires great root and sensitivity. It requires going under an opponent and floating him up so that he loses his contact with the ground. Deprived of his root and striving not to fall, he is unable to hurt us. Battling like water also requires the ability to sense an opponent's center—that place from which he issues power—and thereby recognize where his attacks are coming so as to neutralize them before they are fully realized. Last, battling like water asks us to get behind an opponent's force so that rather than meeting it head-on we can skillfully assist it in the direction it wishes to go, adding a spiral here and there and getting out of the way of his inevitable collapse.

Achieving these goals may be the fullest physical manifestation of our tai chi practice, but it requires a calm, centered, wuji mind. Tai chi's truths are ineluctable. If we seek a deep spiritual system that will open our mind to unfamiliar people, places, things and events while teaching us to see patterns, links and trends, then authentic, martial tai chi is just the thing. When we come in contact with a training partner or opponent whom we cannot handle according to tai chi principles, we have a barometer for our progress; tai chi relentlessly reveals precisely those areas of our mind, body, and life that need work.

THE RELEVANCE OF WEAPONS TRAINING

While casual tai chi players employ only flat shoes, loose clothes, and sometimes soothing music in their pursuit of better balance, relaxation, and health, serious players need serious tools to unlock tai chi's mysteries and secrets. Traditional tai chi weapons do the trick, not because any of us expect to go into battle with them, but because each weapon in the traditional arsenal did and does develop specific tai chi skills. These skills are immediately translatable to weaponless practice, and also to everyday conflict resolution and stress management.

Because they extend our reach, weapons also serve as magnifying glasses, helping us discern errors of alignment, timing, and footwork that we might otherwise not notice. If the relationship between a step and a strike is not quite right, for instance, we can practice for years without seeing or feeling the error. Put a spear, a pole, a halberd, or a long sword in our hand, however, and we'll bang our knee if we step incorrectly, or find ourselves without cover against the attack of a real training partner or imagined foe.

Because weapons add weight and resistance to our training, they teach us not only to relax more deeply (if we don't we may tire prematurely during a practice session) but also to relax in the right places. Sore shoulders, cramped hands, tightness across the upper back, and a stiff neck are just some of the possible consequences of failing to really sink and move like water—inward, downward, and backward with every weapon technique.

Weapons also teach us a great deal about distance. This is important, because without conventional sparring sessions, understanding the role of distance in applying tai chi can be difficult. The need to calculate whether we can reach an opponent with our weapon (or whether our opponent can reach us) introduces a whole new level of complexity to our practice. This complexity challenges our brain to make calculations that may be conscious, even laborious at first, but will eventually become automatic. In doing so, our tai chi "processor" grows more sophisticated and capable.

Last but not least, weapons help our focus. At first, we are simply forced to pay closer attention to our movements so as to master a new routine, learn new specific movements, and not to bang our ear or shin. Later, we must learn to increase the level of our awareness so that our attention can leave the weapon and extend to our empty hand (if we are using a short weapon) and then to the rest of our body. Training with weapons is a great aid to our concentration. Practicing weapons forms and sparring is likely to provide a legitimate shortcut to a wuji state of mind.

THE MAGNIFICENT STRAIGHT SWORD

The sword has a place in world history that transcends military culture. Seen as the symbol of might, purity, lineage, truth, and more, it is also the first weapon most people encounter when learning tai chi, and the one most commonly associated with the art. I have always regarded practicing with a sword to be a method of cutting the bonds that restrain us from being all that we want to be.

The emperor of Chinese blades is the double-edged sword, or jian. Made in large size for a two-handed hold and regular size for a single-hand grip, the jian is a thrusting (stabbing) rather than a cutting weapon. Considered by some as the soul of Chinese martial arts, it began life as a heavy sword designed to penetrate battle armor and has evolved into a lightweight, elegant blade historically popular with educated gentlemen. Training with it builds strength in the wrist, teaches the gauging of distance and coordination of hand and eye, and cultivates relaxation of the arm and shoulder. One reason it is introduced first in the tai chi weapons curriculum is that mastering it takes a lifetime of study, so the sooner we start, the better.

Because it is light and slender, the jian in motion lacks the club-like momentum of heavier weapons. It can be manipulated deftly in the hand, showing up even our subtlest errors like a three-foot-long neon sign. We can feel a great deal through so agile a blade, and we can project our intention and energy (our yi and qi) through it as well. As is true with that other traditional Chinese tool of self-expression, the calligraphy brush, in order to make the blade do our bidding we must move the jian from the waist and hips, all the while keeping our grip loose enough to allow the spiraling movements of reeling silk. While other tai chi weapons are typically performed at speed, the jian, like the open hand form, may be done slowly and with great attention to detail. In the hands of a true master, this most sublime and beautiful instrument seems to float as weightlessly as a soft cloud.

I remember running through the straight sword form in the park one morning with Master Yan when a butterfly alit on the tip of my outstretched sword.

"Please tell me what it means," I implored, barely daring to breathe as the insect alternately opened and closed its wings. "It must be an important omen of some kind."

"It means the butterfly is tired and needs a place to rest," my master replied with barely a hint of a smile. "The trees are too high and the ground is too low but the tip of your sword is just right."

Sharp steel may improve our focus, but it also imperils our noses, ears, elbows, and knees. Thus, we typically begin our practice with a wooden version of this weapon. First, we learn solo exercises, progressing to a form, and then continuing on to tai chi fencing, or "sticking swords." The quality of the sword we use makes little difference when we begin our training, but as we gain experience and skill we should have as good a jian as we can possibly afford. The proper balance, weight, and feel—particularly when we execute explosive, vibrating movements with the blade—are a valuable source of feedback as we try to relax and increase our speed and control of the weapon. Jian are typically manufactured in carbon steel in China, although some domestic bladesmiths offer custom, folded, patterned (Damascus) steel examples at a higher price. Blade lengths range from twenty-eight to thirty-two inches—longer for the two-handed variety.

One particular insight that becomes apparent from training with swords is that the notion of rhythm in fighting is overrated and perhaps even dangerous. Remember, we must always be wary of deception and surprise in combat, and in tai chi we must also avoid attachments and plans. Despite the lull and pull that rhythmic movement promises, setting up a rhythm in fighting makes us predictable and therefore vulnerable. In sword fighting, sparring, Pushing Hands, and form practice, we must watch ourselves carefully and remember to be intuitive, soft, relaxed, and always willing to follow our opponent no matter where she goes.

THE BROADSWORD AND CUTTING SKILL

Learning the curved sword or knife, Dao is typically follows studying the jian in a traditional tai chi curriculum. A far cruder instrument, the Dao resembles a machete and is similarly utilitarian, being a devastating cutting tool even in the hands of new army conscripts. The Dao's slicing attacks are often tied to jumps, leaps, and spins, and train the movements of the hips while developing the torso power that effective cutting requires. When used in a pair, Shuan Dao, these short swords encourage the mind to operate both hands independently—a skill absolutely critical to martial competence yet one dangerous in the learning, as the risk to earlobes, nose, kneecaps, and elbows doubles. Accordingly, I often recommend wooden facsimiles until the student develops a safe level of skill.

In addition to form practice and sparring, the advanced tai chi practitioner will find great benefit in learning to cut well with bladed weapons. Serious cutting requires a serious sword, more often made of carbon steel than stainless. Using a sharp blade on a target such as bamboo, rolled newspaper, or tatami mats—or even better going to a wooded area to sparingly and judiciously find natural botanical targets—can provide some of the best training available. Slicing through targets such as hardwood or bamboo refines the decreasing radius circle (the sword starts a distance from the body but ends up closer to it) essential to high-level cutting.

The immediate feedback to be found in cutting also disciplines the development of a relaxed upper body, integrates the top and bottom of our body, and develops a powerful core. Some people feel that the act of cutting is more than it appears, that when we combine intention and skill and make a cut something special is going on at a level we may not completely understand. Quantum physics may be involved, or some other kind of arcane energetics. Whatever the future scientific explanation for this impression, it contributes to the act of cutting in ways that some tai chi players greatly appreciate.

GENERAL GUAN'S MIGHTY BLADE

Sixteenth generation Chen family member Chen Wang Ting was a garrison commander noted for employing strategies that defeated forces far greater than his own. When formulating an early version of tai chi, Wang Ting drew not only upon his knowledge of Lao Tzu's

Taoist philosophy, but also upon his knowledge of the battlefield weapons of the day. The most influential weapon in the creation of tai chi was a curved sword (Dao) comprised of a two-foot blade on a five-foot shaft. Known to the West as the halberd, it was named both the Spring and Autumn Broadsword or the Guan Dao, both names in reference to the legendary General Guan Yu (died 219 AD)—a warrior so vaunted he was elevated to the rank of a god. Statues of General Guan decorate Chinese restaurants and martial arts schools all over the world, always facing the front door to offer protection to those inside.

Bareback on a horse, knees tucked in, reins in one hand, Guan Dao in the other, the seventeenth century Chinese warrior must have made quite a picture as he cut a swath through the opposing infantry, taking heads and torsos and legs with a blade weighing anywhere between thirty and seventy lbs. As modern tai chi players, we would do well to imagine such a soldier: the powerful legs and core, the mobile hips, the strong waist, the well-developed arms, the way both horse and weapon were managed by sinking, turning, and relaxing.

In traditional Chen style tai chi curriculum, the Guan Dao is taught after learning the first open hand routine, achieving some skill at Pushing Hands and joint locking, and after gaining competence in the straight sword and broadsword. As a result, many beginning players either don't know it exists or don't believe it to be a tai chi weapon. Even so, it is very important and helpful to learn and understand this sword, and counter to convention I often put lightweight wooden versions in the hands of students just starting out, as they find it very helpful in understanding tai chi stances, relaxation and circles.

When my teacher told me I was ready to learn it I was ecstatic, at least in part because I had seen these exotic long swords brandished by wispily bearded heroes in shimmering silk robes in so many 1970s Shaw Brothers Hong Kong martial arts movies. The moment I had a chance, I ordered an inexpensive model from a mail order supply house. When it arrived I immediately took it to my teacher and asked him to show me what the tai chi Guan Dao is all about. The Chen family Guan Dao form is a long one, and I watched, entranced, as my teacher performed about half of it.

"Now you," he said, handing me the weapon.

It felt wonderful in my hand, and I set about duplicating the movements he had performed. When I finished, he stared at me. "I didn't know you could repeat a form after seeing it just one time," he said.

"I didn't know either."

"You're a tai chi genius," he declared. "Do it again."

Warmed by the compliment and excited by the form, I assumed the starting position, and…

Froze. No matter how hard I tried, I could not remember a single move. The second on the wall clock swept around, but still I remained rooted in place.

"Ha," said my teacher, only half in jest. "You're a tai chi idiot."

Having fallen from genius to idiot in less than a minute, I was crushed.

"Do you know what happened?" he demanded.

I shrugged.

"Your mind got in the way."

This was the first of many valuable lessons I, and my students, have learned from studying the Guan Dao. In a way, it makes sense to learn tai chi in the same order it came into being, that is starting with the weapons that inspired the early practitioners and then moving on from there. Perhaps in the future more beginners will be taught this way.

OTHER TAI CHI WEAPONS

In the next chapter I will discuss the various styles of tai chi and the families from which they derive their names. At this point let me say only that each of these family styles relies upon weapons practice to a greater or lesser degree. The Chen family style in which I have been trained features the greatest number of traditional kung fu weapons. These include the three swords already discussed (Guan Dao, Jian, and Dan Dao), the spear, Qiang, the long wooden pole Da Gan, paired short metal cudgels (called Jian like the straight sword, but rendered by a different Chinese character), double hooks, Shuan Gou, short wooden staff, wolf tooth mace (a long shaft with a ball of metal spines on the end) and more.

Each weapon teaches a different set of skills. The spear, for example, is one of the original long weapons of Chinese martial arts and, because of the tactical reach it affords, was of great importance on the battlefield. The spear teaches us both accuracy and projection of power; many consider it the heart of Chinese kung fu. Because it involves jumping, leaping, and low stances, spear fighting requires strong legs. Its small, efficient, martially precise movements also make great demands upon the torso, arms, wrists, and hands. Any student who spends time on proper spear techniques soon learns the critical importance of both precision and relaxation, as the length of the spear magnifies errors and upper body tension, making fine maneuvers very challenging.

As is common to most tai chi forms, movements in the spear forms typically have poetic names such as Iron Bull Plows the Field (Tie Niu Geng Di) and Green Dragon Extends its Claws (Qing Long Xian Zhua). The derivation of the spear movements in tai chi extends back into antiquity and borrows from other fighting systems. Spear techniques emphasize sticking to our opponent's spear in much the way we stick together during Pushing Hands practice. The result is that one rarely hears the clacking sound of wood against wood typical of spear exchanges in other kung fu styles. Instead, tai chi spear training focuses on using efficient spirals to disarm and attack in a single move.

Many of the same comments can be made of the long pole, Da Gan, a traditional tai chi weapon whose use predates even the spear.

Typically made of eight–ten feet of white Chinese wax wood, training with the long pole requires a unique combination of relaxation and upper body strength. The pole develops our forearms, too, and teaches us a whip-like, explosive rotation of the body's core that shakes the weapon in spectacular fashion, producing penetrating deflections and thrusts.

The specific qualities of each weapon aside, the most important thing to remember is to keep our equilibrium and extend our intelligence into the metal and the wood. Rather than "becoming the sword," an exhortation common to other martial arts, in tai chi we want the sword (or other weapon) to become us. The notion that we would want to subjugate a finely tuned martial arts practitioner rife with experience, sensitivity, creativity, and passion to an unconscious, inanimate piece of metal flies in the face of tai chi's essence. Whenever we have a weapon in our hand, that weapon should brim with the vibrancy of our practice.

EXPLORATIONS

The explorations below offer a taste of tai chi's self-defense techniques. Of course we cannot actually master any dimension of tai chi from a book, but we can start to learn some of the basic concepts here. These exercises are designed to serve as a jumping off point for further work with a qualified teacher in a group class setting. There is no substitute for hours of devoted practice, particularly with a wide range of cooperative training partners.

Waving Hands Like Clouds

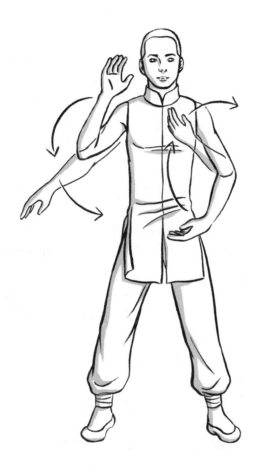

DESPITE THE FACT THAT TAI CHI APPEARS COMPLEX TO THE untrained eye, all the system's spiraling movements are concocted from a combination of simple circles. These circles are dictated by basic human anatomy. In the first and second explorations we will explore some ways to circle with the arms.

Begin with your right hand positioned palm up, fingers relaxed but together, just below your navel. Raise the hand along the midline of the body, fingertips up. When you pass the level of your head, turn the hand so that the palm rotates outward. Now extend the hand so that the movement proscribes a large circle and then turn it so that the fingertips point downward. Continue the downward circle of the arm until the hand returns to where it began, just below the navel. Broadly, the motion has a scooping quality, as if you are bringing something up toward your mouth and then turning your hand to throw it away.

To make sure you understand the plane in which you are circling your arms, which is parallel to the front of your body, imagine that you are standing face toward the wall in a narrow alley between two buildings. There is little room in front or in back so the circle must stay close to the plane of your body, never extending too far in front of you, and not at all behind. This circle, in combination with the turn of the arm around its axis, creates a three-dimensional spiraling motion. Remember to keep your elbow pointed downward and your shoulders relaxed all the way through. After you are comfortable performing the motion with each hand individually, you can try moving the hands together so as to create a windmill effect. To begin a double circle, your right hand may start high up and the left hand low and then, circling, exchange positions. At first it may be challenging to keep both hands moving because your attention naturally jumps from one hand to the other, and when it leaves a hand, that hand freezes. Knowing this, try your best to keep things moving. After a few sessions, you should start to get the hang of it.

Try to remain relaxed while doing this movement. Don't hold your breath. If your shoulders become tense or sore, take a break, but try to repeat the last version, with both arms moving, over and over again for five–ten minutes, treating the exploration like a meditation. During the course of a few weeks of daily practice sessions, it can become hypnotically relaxing to think only of your relaxed hands and your circling arms. This movement is called "Waving Hands Like Clouds" because it should feel light and graceful.

Rolling Arms Backward

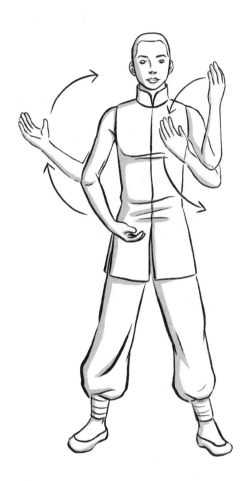

ONCE YOU HAVE MASTERED THE "UP THE MIDDLE" CIRCLE, IT is time to try its opposite. This qualifies for a separate exploration because human anatomy dictates it be quite a different movement. Keeping your shoulders down and relaxed when circling up the middle is a simple matter. When you circle your arms so that your hands come down the centerline of your body, however, your shoulders are necessarily engaged. Engaging your waist to assist in the movement helps to keep the shoulders from rising too much.

Once again, start circling your arms in front of you, pretending that you are sandwiched between two walls. The hand position as the arm descends the midline of the body has the fingertips up and the palm pointed away from center as it goes down. As in the previous exercise, the bottom of the circle is just below the navel and the top of the circle is as high above the head as you can make it while still keeping an overall round shape to the movement. As before, once you can do this circle with each hand individually, try doing both hands at the same time, again being patient with your brain as it learns to move both arms at the same time. As is the case for the preceding exercise, this one will become quite meditative and relaxing—while developing sensitivity in the hands and circling skills—if practiced for five–ten minutes a day for some weeks. Once you have enjoyed circling in both directions for a month or so, you are ready for the next exploration.

EXPLORATION #3

Rabbit and Hunter

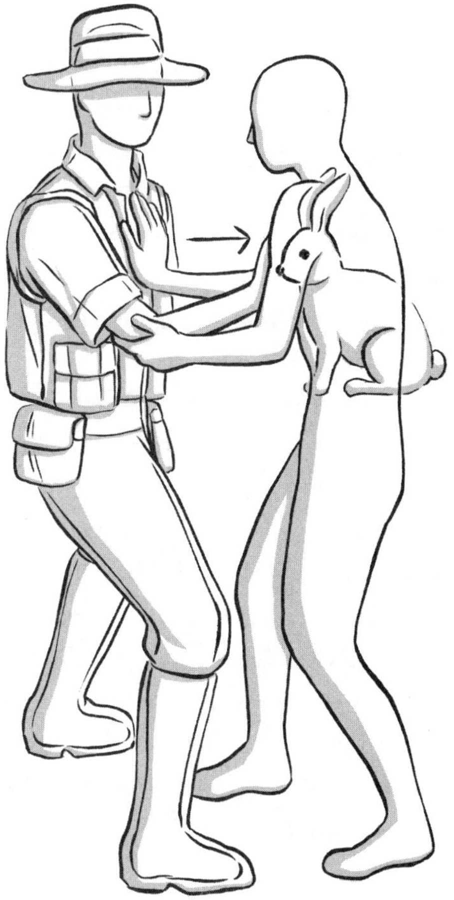

THIS TWO-PERSON EXPLORATION IS A TAI CHI GAME THAT BUILDS on the skills developed in the previous chapters. To begin, stand facing a willing and cooperative partner of approximately your own height. Now step forward to the right front corner as your partner does the same. Your feet should be right beside each other. Now put your right hand on your partner's breastbone as she puts hers on yours. Cup your left hand under your partner's left elbow.

One of you (you will switch roles shortly) now assumes the role of the rabbit, while the other assumes the role of the hunter. The hunter is the person using the fingers and palms of both hands to seek what information they can about the other's center of gravity. This means she is gently sensing and even slightly pushing to see how her partner can evade her force. The rabbit is the person moving away from the force by sinking, turning, spiraling until she loses her balance.

This is a game of very subtle movements, not big shoves. It's a co-operative, following game aimed at learning to sense, and then pursue, another person's center of gravity. Emphasizing on listening and feeling, this exercise draws on the sensitivity drills that have come before. Done properly, all your movements in this exploration should be light, slow, gentle, and truly explorative. When one of you loses your balance it is because you have reached the lower limits of your imaginary rabbit warren—in other words you have run out of room to turn or sink or evade the relentless push of your partner's hand.

There are no precise moves to make in this exploration, as there have been in previous, because each session is completely creative and unique. The only rule is that you must use light touch rather than brute force. Avoid having a plan as you follow and you will do so more successfully. In turn, each of you will discover—and then defeat—that combination of breath, muscular tension, balance, gravity and flexibility that is required to remain upright.

Tai Chi's Unique
Combative Flavor

Martial encounters universally involve an exchange: one fighter attacks, another defends. This pugilistic conversation occurs in all the world's martial arts, including American boxing, French Savate, Indonesian Penjat Silat, Filipino Kali, Japanese Karate, Russian Special Forces Systema, Mongolian wrestling, Israeli Krav Maga, Chinese Kung Fu, Hawaiian Kaihewalu Lua, and more. Fighter A does one thing, Fighter B counters; first a punch, then a block; first a kick, then a dodge; first a grab, then a trap. Such a contentious rhythm is the stuff of combat—bred in the bone of the true fighter and even inculcated into those of us with the modest desire to defend ourselves from chance encounters.

Tai chi is the sole exception to this rule, the only martial art in the world in which such an exchange does not take place. Indeed, seeing herself and her opponent as a unified system, the tai chi player must be free of the instinct to give and to take. If she is born with it, she must subdue it; if she has been trained to it, she must make every effort to lose that training. Instead, she must attach to no particular strategy or technique; her highest mental goal is simply to maintain "wuji" (emotional equilibrium) while her sole physical goal is to maintain the unrestricted flow of life force, qi, required by optimal health.

If, in the course of protecting this calm and this flow, an aggressor goes flying or suffers grievous damage, it is not because we have any such intention. Purely speaking, tai chi is a consummately self-centered (but not selfish) art. A tai chi player's sole intention must be to use such concepts as harmony, balance, relaxation, softness, and rooting to create sophisticated, spiraling techniques that preserve, protect, defend, and restore her equilibrium. The tai chi player never thinks, worries, or plans what to do with an attack, nor does she play catch-up to an opponent's gambit. Where the opponent may rely upon deception, she must remain clear-headed and relaxed, responding but never reacting, always flowing along the path of least resistance, maximal efficiency, and best martial effect.

The fact that tai chi is often portrayed first and foremost as a health practice—and that its moves are soft and slow and often lack obvious punches and kicks—lead some fighters to doubt the art's martial effectiveness. Once we understand tai chi's unique orientation, however, we find profound combat training at work. Tai chi changes our body and mind in fundamental ways. Its slow moves help us discover our weak spots, eliminate our bad habits, forge a strong mind-body link, condition us to never meet force with force, and help an opponent use his energy against himself. Combining defense and offense into single maneuvers, tai chi players become lightning fast fighters, neither easily deceived by sneak tactics nor overwhelmed by greater force. The general strategy is to use joint locking, qinna, to deprive an opponent of his balance and then follow up with appropriate fajing strikes to finish the conflict.

Tai chi is not purely defensive. In addition to devastating strikes and locks and effectively borrowing their opponents' force, tai chi players generate their own bullwhip-like power by combining relaxation, spiral movements, and the force of gravity. Contrasted with the famous one-inch punch of Chinese film star Bruce Lee, high-level tai chi fighters are capable of what we might call a no-inch punch. Once mastered, this technique has a penetrating quality and can be performed with no apparent windup, leaving the punching hand in contact with the target the whole time. It need not be expressed only with a fist, but can be done as an open-palm strike or even a jerk downward. Eventually, kicks can be performed this way, too, as can head butts, knee, elbow, and torso strikes. The tai chi master player is like a bomb, ready to go off right at the spot where it is attacked, yet otherwise cool, calm, and relaxed.

Pushing Hands

ANYONE WHO HAS EVER BEEN IN A REAL STREET FIGHT WILL tell you that two things are universally true. One is that the distances at which competitors stand in karate and kung fu tournaments are unrealistic, the other is that most fights end up on the ground. What street toughs know is that in order to have a real and decisive effect on our opponent—namely to do what is necessary to end the conflict—we can't stand at a gentlemanly distance and throw speculative kicks and sportsmanlike jabs. We have to get in close enough to hit our man. That means being in close enough to be hit in return.

This news is of no concern to wrestlers or Mixed Martial Arts (MMA) fighters, and not much concern to Western-style boxers either, as these fighting styles are comfortable with close-quarter combat. So is tai chi. While it remains true that most players are primarily interested in promoting their health and well-being, a safe and effective method of training combat contact is built into the very core of the system. This method is called "pushing hands" ("sensing hands" might actually be a better name) and although when practiced with an inappropriately competitive attitude or done with an excess of enthusiasm it can become a bit unruly, it is properly executed as a cooperative, learning experience.

At its core, pushing hands teaches us to rely on our structure and design to accept a force—a grab, strike, kick, lock, push, or shove—

without losing either our physical alignment or our emotional equilibrium. Moving with equal ease in all directions and wasting no energy on organic friction or drag, we return any attack as close as possible to the point at which we receive it. This requires great sensitivity, a skill the tai chi classics (a collection of treatises written over a period of hundreds of years) exhort us to develop to the point where we can know an opponent's next move before he does. In pushing hands the two players create a single energetic, intentional unit. The highest skill is to return the force we receive precisely at the point of contact.

Success in pushing hands safely also builds experience, confidence, comfort with contact, and the ability to discover an opponent's weaknesses. It also develops rooting, three-dimensional movement, relaxation, alignment, smooth transfer of balance, and perhaps most importantly of all, a creative and unflappable mind. Regardless of why we practice tai chi, pushing hands practice represents an essential way to build your sensitivity and test your root. It is an indispensable skill that will bring your tai chi to life.

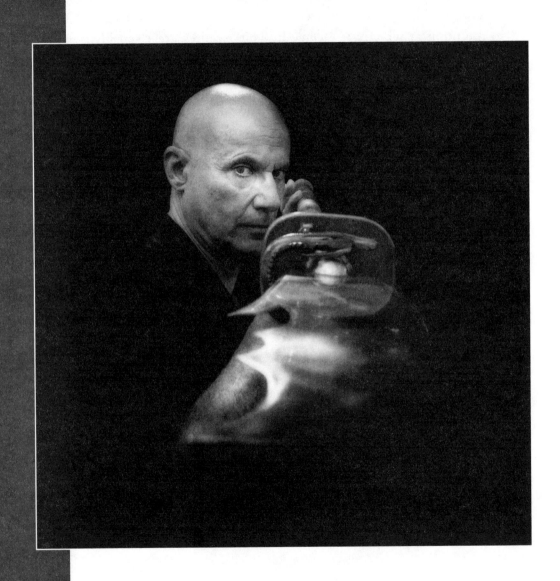

"To be always talking is against nature. For the same reason a hurricane never lasts a whole morning, nor a rainstorm all day."

TAO TE CHING, V. 23, (ARTHUR WALEY, TRANSLATOR)

TEACHERS, TRADITIONS, CLASSES, AND TOOLS

Here in the West, we have suffered from a disproportionate emphasis on logic and rational thought for centuries, in many quarters deriding intuition and emotion as mere distractions. The explosion of interest in tai chi in the West may be a sign that we are ready to abandon the idea of humans as computers and re-establish a balanced interaction between rational thought and intuition, between logic and emotion, and between what we have long considered to be a divided body and mind. What we get from tai chi is not a blind obedience to intuition, but a refinement of that intuition to the point where it is very much trustworthy.

Any worthy hobby, sport, or passion gives us a context within which to test ourselves and to grow. Tai chi's methods are exceptionally brilliant, battle-tested, ancient, and wise, but the art's real value is that rather than teach us to hit a ball a great distance or jump with agility, tai chi reveals how to take advantage of natural forces with the least effort and the most result. In short, tai chi teaches us about life.

PRACTICE

There is only one thing we must do to glean the marvelous benefits of tai chi, and that is to practice. Practice is where history, philosophy, science, tradition, body mechanics, energetics, martial experience, mindfulness, and self-awareness come together. It is our refuge from the hustle and bustle of our everyday life and it is our laboratory for self-inquiry and self-cultivation. As an established system with a long history, tai chi has various tools that we can use to manage our stress, creatively express ourselves, quiet our mind, gain strength and flexibility, achieve martial competence, and live a long and healthy life.

The first and foremost of those tools is called the tai chi form. As mentioned in the introduction, the form is a sequence of movements (also called postures) strung together like pearls. Each move has a specific benefit from the point of view of Traditional Chinese Medicine, and as such represents a balance between yin and yang in the body. Requiring relaxation and repetition to achieve, each move also represents a range of possible martial application. Beginning, intermediate, and advanced forms are the backbone of nearly all Asian fighting systems, and are tailored to teach traditional weapons as well. The forms in tai chi are some of the longest and most complex in any martial art.

In addition to being a culture obsessed with keeping records (thus providing a rich, verifiable history of one of the world's greatest cultures) the Chinese put great stock in numerology and have certain numbers they associate with good fortune, special occasions, and power. One hundred and eight is a particularly auspicious number in many ancient cultures, and is the number of postures in the authentic, original, long forms of many tai chi styles. Fifty-four (half of one hundred and eight) can be the number of movements of shorter forms. Thirteen is another auspicious number and designates the so-called tai chi postures. The first eight of the tai chi thirteen denote energies derived from the eight trigrams (a traditional description of reality in Taoist cosmology) and the last five are steps that correspond to the five elements of nature (earth, metal, water, fire, and wood), key concepts in Traditional Chinese Medicine. The thirteen postures listed below are incorporated into the forms of a variety of tai chi styles, each of which interprets them differently. Note that the first four have been explained more fully in Chapter 3 and are included here for the sake of completeness.

- Peng (ward-off)
- Liu (roll-back)
- Ji (press)
- An (push)
- Tsai (split)
- Lieh (change direct)
- Zhou (elbow)
- Cao (shoulder strike)
- Jin Bu (advance)
- Tui Bu (retreat)
- Zuo Ku (step left)
- You Pan (step right)
- Zhong Ting (maintain a central position)

The number thirteen also represents the principles of tai chi, which are:

- Sink the shoulders and drop the elbows.
- Relax the chest and round the back.
- Sink the qi down to the Dantian.
- Gently lift the head.
- Relax the waist and hips.
- Differentiate between empty and full/weighted and unweighted/yin and yang.
- Properly coordinate the top and bottom halves of the body.
- Use insight rather than brute force.
- Harmonize the inside of the body with the external world.

- Let the yi (intention) lead the qi (energy).
- Cultivate wuji (stillness) of mind.
- Incorporate wuji (stillness) in motion.
- Move evenly and continuously throughout the form.

Ultimately, tai chi principles and movements are simple, if not easy. Form practice allows us to test our understanding of the postures and principles long before we need them to fight a parking lot assailant or chronic disease. When we practice forms, sometimes we start at the beginning and keep going until we have done every move we know. Sometimes we pick a "piece" of tai chi and do it over and over again, relishing doing it just a bit better than we did before, all the while sinking, turning, and relaxing.

Listening to our body during practice is essential. We should notice small changes and rejoice in them, and we should recognize our cycles, enjoy our plateaus, and rejoice in our advances. If we want to use tai chi to connect our mind and body we must apply every shred of our attention to the practice. No thinking about motorcycling through New Zealand, shopping every mall in Paris, or yearning to watch the home game on a big screen with a beer in our hand. No thinking about what's for lunch, coveting a neighbor's sports car, or planning a beach picnic. Tai chi requires that we be completely present. When we are, we burn new, hot wires from our brain to our body and back—pathways along which new information flows in fresh ways.

Learning tai chi is much like being abroad in a wondrous, exotic land. The signs are often unintelligible and the landmarks strange. Traveling, we must be creative and use whatever maps and tools we can (our forms, prescribed sequences of tai chi movements, are an example) ever mindful to step lightly, navigate deftly, and be patient with ourselves. We won't get anywhere by being bullheaded. Intelligence must replace compulsivity. Discipline must include patience. We must be sensitive to the fact that our mindbody has its own timetable for learning rooting, relaxation, silk reeling, meditation, Dantian rotation, and more. Our teachers, classes, and our training partners represent investments in growth and healing; we must choose them carefully.

In our attempts to "master" the art, we may confuse knowing many facts, techniques, or tai chi trivia with being able to do tai chi. We may embrace the world of virtual tai chi—a trap in this endeavor as it is in so many others—and waste our time watching tai chi videos online rather than practicing forms, pushing hands, or meditation. If we do get up and move we may become form collectors, learning one set of movements after another like dance steps while never going deep inside to our still places and feeling our qi circulate, our blood move, our intention manifest, our heart and joints open. Such collecting is not fruitful; in tai chi it is better to relinquish goals in favor of experience, and the destination in favor of the journey.

ETIQUETTE

Bringing tai chi into your life means embracing new ideas and a long-standing martial culture. Taoist sages, warriors, and monks have used the art to condition their bodies, strengthen their spirit, and transform their minds for hundreds, perhaps thousands of years. Millions of everyday people—bound together only by their desire to fill their lives with meaning and their bodies with strength, health, and energy—continue to follow suit. Out of respect for this tradition, martial etiquette offers some guidelines to follow at tai chi class. This wu de (pronounce it woo duh) tells us to address our instructor as Sifu (pronounce it shir-foo or sea-foo) as we would an honored uncle or father. The term implies not merely respect for the teacher but a bond of loyalty and responsibility that flows both ways. Honoring our teachers means honoring all those who brought this wonderful art to us, as well as honoring our own commitment to self-betterment. The sifu, in turn, accepts responsibility for our learning and for our well-being, too.

There are always exceptions (as when players know each other very well) but as a general rule in a traditional martial arts setting it is more accepted to bow than to shake hands, clap each other on the shoulder, hug, etc. The nuanced subject of traditional bows could easily fill a book dedicated to that subject alone, but in tai chi simply making a fist with the right hand, knuckles up, and then folding the left hand over it, also knuckles up, is generally appropriate. Holding the hands at the level of the sternum and a bit away from the body is a fine gesture of respect. In fact, in China this bow is used not only by monks and fighters, but is a common everyday greeting, particularly among the older generation.

Most tai chi teachers try to set a class tone that reflects the underlying values the art advances and the culture it represents. This is not an American art, and is not a place where mainstream American culture obtains. Using a cell phone to text or hold a conversation while a teacher is talking may have become everyday behavior in many school classrooms, but is a no-no in tai chi class. So is offering opinions when they have not been solicited and practicing on your own when you are part of a group that is supposed to be working together on a particular skill.

It is appropriate to show respect for students who have been there longer than you have, if only to acknowledge their hard work. In most martial arts schools, and some tai chi classes, too, students line up to bow to the teacher at the beginning and end of class, often organizing themselves, according to level, from the most senior and proficient to the least. This is useful and important because unlike in some other martial arts there are no rank belts in tai chi, so sometimes the only way we know who best to watch or ask for help is by seeing where they stand in line.

Asking questions is far more acceptable in the West than it is in the East—where the assumption is that the teacher has your best interests at heart and knows exactly why he or she is asking you to do something—but some younger Chinese teachers have learned to adapt. China is not a democracy and tai chi class is not typically a democracy either. Implicit in the nature of the class is that the teacher has some valuable information that we would really like to learn, and we want to be respectful of both the information itself and the years of effort the teacher has put in to master something that is quite special and hard-won. Most tai chi teachers hope that we will be patient with the process and hold our questions long enough to let the answers unfold.

Visiting masters, particularly if they are from China, really expect us to be sufficiently knowledgeable to pose meaningful queries that cannot easily be answered by other students or teachers with less experience. This can seem daunting sometimes, but there are two sides to it. While poorly informed questions are not appreciated, good ones are treasured and will light up a good teacher like a chandelier. If we are not sure that what we are asking is substantial and important, it may be better not to ask it right away.

Making the effort to understand tai chi etiquette shows that we respect the history and tradition behind the art. Such a showing is a sign of respect not only to those who have come before and striven to develop an amazing system of personal development, but also a sign of respect to ourselves and our own efforts. What worked centuries ago to keep things cool between rival teachers, factions, or martial styles works today to generate warmth and camaraderie inside the school. Treating our classmates with affection and respect is beneficial because sooner or later we will reach a stage in our training where we embark on two-person exercises. When this happens, we will profit greatly from a cooperative spirit, and from keeping competition to a minimum. The Golden Rule must be in force. In tai chi two heads and two sets of arms and legs are often more helpful, if not better, than one.

CLASSES

While tai chi is not yet as common as yoga here in the West, it certainly shares many aspects with that practice: it requires no specialized equipment—at least at the beginning—is relatively inexpensive, increasingly popular, and can be done either in limited indoor quarters or in a salubrious outdoor setting. Tai chi's stress-busting benefits seem to be the primary reason most people adopt the practice, although the spectacular tai chi segment of the opening ceremonies at the 2008 Beijing Olympic Games certainly introduced the art to television audiences all over the world.

Throughout East Asia, tai chi classes can be found in public parks and in the backyard training halls of well-known teachers. Here in the U.S. we are more likely to find classes at gyms, recreational halls, and martial arts schools, as well as at hospitals and senior centers. Most players find classes by word of mouth or by doing an Internet search for teachers in their local area. There are typically between ten and twenty students in a class, though some classes may have more or fewer students than that. Some teachers require a monthly commitment; others favor a pay-per-class option. Costs at the time of this writing typically run between $10 and $20 per session, although master teachers command higher prices and some classes in parks may be free.

Classes usually last between sixty–ninety minutes and often begin with a standard warm-up sequence (frequently a qigong set like the Eight Pieces of Brocade) followed by gentle stretching. Form practice comes next, with the class working as a unit or, if the program has been in place long enough for students to achieve more, groups of students breaking off to practice according to their level. Weapons practice and Pushing Hands training often occur at the end of the session.

On the surface it would seem that trying a class before signing up is the best way to determine if it is right for us, but this may be less true of tai chi than it is of other exercises. Tai chi is such a different experience than other exercise classes that I explain to beginners that the one quality that most assures success in the art (and by success I mean that we find life to be better with tai chi than without it) has nothing to do with nationality, flexibility, fitness, strength, or martial experience. That single most important quality, rather, is being able to make bewildering our friend. The first few classes will indeed be baffling, often rife with unfamiliar words and always with unfamiliar movements. It also very much helps to turn off any self-critical program we may tend to run in our head. Chastising ourselves for not learning faster or giving in to competitive feelings while watching others around us will only slow our progress, or worse, lead us to give up before we even get started. The class that is the most initially inviting, therefore, may not in the end be the one that is best for us. Even so, when you find a class that seems to suit you, consider making a three-month commitment to the teacher. If you are new to the art, it will take you that long to really get a feel and a satisfying taste of the art.

If we are highly stressed or ill and hoping that tai chi will "fix" us, or if we have studied for a long time and feel we can truly benefit from our teacher's undivided attention, we may opt for a private class. In some parts of this country such lessons may, at the time of this writing, be had for as little as $30/session, although well-known teachers and famous masters may charge far more. Some teachers may be amenable to teaching a "semi-private" for two or three individuals so as to help defray costs. Private instruction typically lasts between thirty–sixty minutes, and as in so many other areas of life, we get what we pay for.

There simply is no substitute for having a knowledgeable master correct our mistakes and steer us in the right direction. A typical scenario might be to attend group class once, twice, or three times a week, and to have a private lesson either once a week, once a month, or at a frequency somewhere in between.

Years ago I came into Master Yan's school one day and found him teaching a private class to a young woman I had never seen before. To my surprise, he was teaching her an advanced weapons form—one I myself had yet to learn. I watched her do the movements and was not particularly impressed. When she was gone, I asked my teacher how long she had been training.

"Three months," he answered.

"Are you kidding? I've been training for five years and you still haven't taught me that form!"

Forbearing as ever, Master Yan merely smiled at me. "How far do you want to take your tai chi?" he asked.

"To the moon," I cried. "I love this art so much."

Master Yan nodded. "The girl who just left is a dilettante. Next week, she will be playing tennis. You, on the other hand, want to build a tai chi skyscraper, and for that you need a big foundation. All the time you are spending working on the basic stances, footwork, and forms will stand you in good stead as you go higher and higher with your practice. Now quit worrying about what other people are doing and get to work."

Our early tai chi training is indeed all about foundation. That is why in writer/director David Mamet's film *Redbelt*, the protagonist, a martial arts teacher, tells a new student that the first step in training is the most difficult. "What is the first step?" the new student asks. "Leaving the outside world outside when you step in here," is the answer.

Part of tai chi's magic is that it brings us to a relaxed place and helps us to stay there even after we go home. Once we have found a good class, we will be well served if we stick with it, expanding our experiences with the art by sharing them with others, and by broadening the context in which they apply. Testing the lessons by applying them in every area of life is the whole point of tai chi. Doing so will keep us happy and healthy and young.

TEACHERS

In the old days, tai chi students typically began training at an early age. Most often these were boys, but sometimes girls learned, too.

Some were indentured to the teacher, sweeping the training hall, cleaning the master's home, even working in his fields to guarantee their tuition. Over time, some of these "indoor" students were drafted and went to war. If they were lucky, they came back mortally grateful for the teaching they had received, as it had likely saved their lives. If they were good enough, they became bodyguards or professional soldiers. Later in life they themselves became teachers, preserving the art while using it to train a new generation of fighters as well as to bolster their own health and the health of those close to them.

Throughout the arc of their careers, students were bound to their teacher. They needed guidance, protection, and the very special and unique knowledge he possessed. Sometimes the master's teaching style was severe, but the motivation was nearly always right and good, and the results outstanding. Very rarely did a teacher praise a student—a blow across the back with a bamboo rod was more common than a compliment—but when a compliment did occur, it really meant something.

The teacher, in turn, sought out students who could keep the art alive. He was very circumspect in this process, as years spent training someone who would either misuse the art or never fully grasp the physical or spiritual dimensions were years wasted. To protect his "investment" the teacher became part instructor and part parent to his martial "family," as the title sifu suggests.

These days, we shop for teachers the way we shop for cars or carpets. There are only a few older masters left, and those are often caught between cultures and generations. Usually they are available only for workshops and seminars, as they either travel about or require students to go to see them in China. The good news for those of us who cannot make such a commitment is that a younger generation of tai chi teachers of different backgrounds and nationalities is emerging around the world. These are often passionate and talented players, and are intent on spreading the gospel according to tai chi. They ally themselves with local students, and run good marketing campaigns, too.

Choosing the right teacher is a very personal matter. In some parts of the country we do not have many options, and of course any tai chi teacher is better than no tai chi teacher. In areas where there is a variety of teachers to choose from, we will likely want just the right blend of commerciality and dedication, professionalism, practicality, and support, along with caring, passion, and excellence. Tai chi practice touches all aspects of our life. Accordingly, a teacher's humility, expertise, judgment, restraint, and insight are important both in terms of teaching clearly and in terms of showing that the art has transformed the teacher in the way that we ourselves would like to be transformed. Taking time to talk to the teacher before committing is a must. If she does not have time to talk, go elsewhere. Ask other students what they have gotten from the class, and how they feel about her.

In tai chi, lineage is extremely important. Since the variety of family styles and range of approaches to the art make the existence of any universal and legitimate tai chi accrediting body neither likely nor particularly desirable, the first step in assuring the legitimacy of a teacher is to ask about her lineage. A highly qualified teacher will be proud of that link to the past and be eager to share it. The shorter the list of people between a teacher and a member of a founding family (Chen, Sun, Yang, etc.), the more authentic their command of the art is likely to be. Short lineage lines mean more direct transmission of information and less chance for dilution, loss, and misunderstanding.

If a prospective teacher is vague about her lineage, or if it emerges that she has learned from a video or by attending a variety of workshops, it might be best for us to look elsewhere. A qualified teacher was taught by another qualified teacher. If the teacher we are interviewing does not positively glow with pride and pleasure while discussing her lineage, we must find one who does.

STYLES OF TAI CHI

Although the precise origins of tai chi get murkier the farther back in time we go, what we can confidently say is that tai chi knowledge and wisdom have been passed down through many generations. Over the centuries since Chen Wang Ting (1580–1660) and his collaborators planted the Chen family tai chi tree, quite a few branches have sprouted. Besides Chen style, which persists, the major branches are Yang, Wu/Hao, Wu, Sun, and Zhaobao/Qing Ping. These days, Yang is the most popular style, followed by Wu, Chen, and Sun. Any and all branches and styles are worth learning, and while we can say that certain ones may offer more or less to the martially inclined player, any tai chi style will deepen our mind and strengthen our body. In the end, most people choose a style because it is the one available to them.

Philosophically and spiritually speaking, all styles of tai chi are Taoist practices and thus connect strongly to Lao Tzu's *Tao Te Ching*, to meditation and to a balanced, harmonious diet and lifestyle. Physically, Chen style tai chi is the most athletically demanding, featuring the twisting spirals discussed throughout this book, as well as explosive movements, jumping, leaping, low stances, and heavy weapons. Arm motions can appear snakelike in Chen style, and there is a great emphasis on the three-dimensional rotation of the hips and surrounding muscles, the Dantian. Shifting weight is a particular skill in Chen tai chi, as is the idea of having the upper body move like water.

While the movements may be complex, small, and sometimes subtle, Chen stylists contend that their art's "wringing water from a towel" quality moves qi quite well. As in all tai chi the thigh and gluteal muscles work hard, but perhaps hardest in this style because of the low stances and leaps. There are a number of variants of Chen style tai chi, generally linked to specific lineages within the family. Chenjiaguo, the Chen village, has in recent years become a popular international training destination.

More people practice Yang style tai chi than any other. Legend has it that the style arose when a gifted player, Yang Lu Chan (1799–1872, known as Yang the Invincible), learned Chen style and then simplified it in order to make it more accessible. Chen style's explosive movements, low stances, and emphasis on three-dimensional "silk reeling" are diminished in Yang style, as the emphasis has turned from the system's original martial purpose to health and longevity. Yang style movements are generally obvious and large, the better to encourage the flow of qi in a more straightforward way. Yang style is rarely taught with the same emphasis on weapons as traditional Chen style, and is fully as likely to be found in health clubs, recreational and senior centers, and local parks as it is to be offered in martial arts schools. Due in part to its popularity, there are numerous "strains" of Yang style.

Wu Chuan Yau (1834–1902)—a Manchurian member of the Imperial guard in Beijing—studied with Yang Lu Chan and others to conceive Wu style tai chi. His disciple, Wu Chien Chuan (1870–1942), joined others to create the Beijing Institute of Physical Education, where he refined and popularized the Wu style art. Traditional Wu style training includes an open hand form, a straight sword form, a broadsword form, and a spear form, along with pushing hands and other applications. Visually, Wu style is elegant and spare, with movements typically executed in a higher stance than Chen style, and with obvious leaning of the back and circling of the waist. Overall, the body's frame is smaller in this style than in some others. As in Yang style there is an emphasis on health, and as in Chen style, Wu style trains internal power. Variations on Wu style tai chi include Beijing Wu, Shanghai Wu, and Southeast Asian Wu.

Zhaobao Village is a couple of miles up the road from the Chen Village, and, predictably enough, tai chi practiced there closely resembles traditional Chen style tai chi. Some teachers allege that Zhaobao tai chi can be traced back to an early master named Jiang Fa (1547–1655), a contemporary of Chen Wang Ting who is alternately described as his servant, collaborator, and close friend. Jiang Fa is also allegedly connected to a Taoist monk, perhaps from Wudang Mountain, a cradle of Chinese kung fu. Zhaobao is a style ripe with sweeps, trips, and locks. It is practiced at various heights according to level of mastery, and players pay a great deal of attention to the role of intention (yi) in this system's movements. A pivotal player in this style, Chen Qing Ping (1795–1868) is credited with a great contribution to the development of this particular art, and there are some who follow a style close if not identical to mainstream Zhaobao tai chi. Practitioners may refer to that art as Qing Ping style.

Wu (Hao) style tai chi derives from Wu Yu Hsiang (1813–1880), an upper class scholar who made valuable contributions to tai chi theory. He studied with Yang Lu Chan and briefly with Chen Qing Ping. This style has smaller movements, higher, and simpler (jumps and explosive movements deleted) than the ancestral Chen family form, and emphasizes the balance between yin and yang in motion, and a still, calm mind. While the healthful nature of the practice is stressed in this relatively uncommon form of tai chi, so is careful listening to the opponent's energy and intention.

Neo-Confucianist and Taoist scholar, Sun Lu Tang (1861–1932) was already an expert in two internal martial arts styles related to tai chi—Hsing-I Ch'uan (Mind Boxing) and Baguazhang (8 Trigram Palm)—when he met Wu (Hao) tai chi master Hao Wei Chen (1842–1920). Impressed with Hao's art, Sun combined it with the other two styles he knew to create an exciting new synthesis he named Sun style tai chi. This style is especially aesthetically pleasing because of the spear-oriented, direct, vertical attacks and animal fluidity it incorporates from Hsing-I Ch'uan, and the elegant, circular stepping it incorporates from Baguazhang. Overall, this is a sophisticated and elegant system that often appeals to those of us who have had training in other martial arts and are looking for something different.

We tai chi players tend to be passionate about our art. The deeper our study, the more seriously we tend to take loyalty to our teacher and lineage. As worldwide interest in our art grows, comparisons between styles may become a bit contentious. In my view, it is better to practice than argue. In any other tai chi player we have a kindred spirit, and in any other tai chi style we have a kindred art.

CROSS-TRAINING

In *Drunken Master*, one of his early kung fu films, box office giant, Jackie Chan plays a callow student who endures brutal training at the hands of a perpetually inebriated teacher. Poked with bamboo poles, suspended upside down, forced to repeatedly fill an empty bucket with water, and landing on the back of his wrists while doing push ups to avoid being struck by his teacher's stick, Chan gradually reaches a superlative level of conditioning.

This cinematic rendition of kung fu in earlier times entertainingly makes the excellent point that training is a practical matter. If we have dumbbells, we use dumbbells. If we have bricks, we use bricks. If we have kettle bells, we use kettle bells, and if we have stones we use stones. In the early days, tai chi practice involved weapons of various weights and sizes, and their use provided a complete training system. Integrated into an active lifestyle it provided everything we could possibly need to become healthy, strong, clear-minded, and long lived.

The same is true today, with a very specific caveat. To fully strengthen and train the upper body as well as it does the lower, tai chi requires both Pushing Hands training and weapons practice. The former integrates hand movements with footwork, while the latter builds coordination and muscle tone in the arms, shoulders, back, and chest. Both training tools strengthen the body's core and teach us how to properly rotate the Dantian.

If the tai chi program we have selected does not involve these aspects of the art, either because the teacher is afraid they may be off-putting to some students or because he is not fluent in them, tai chi is not the complete strength-training program it was designed to be. More, since practicing with the straight sword, broadsword, Guan Dao, spear, long pole, iron sticks, wolf tooth mace, or other traditional weapon means lifting weight, dropping into low stances, and explosive jumping and leaping, omitting these training tools means we lose the aerobic benefits of the traditional curriculum.

That is where cross-training comes in. Walking, swimming, cycling, and weight lifting can replace what is missing from an oversimplified tai chi curriculum. Walking is accessible to players at nearly any fitness level and is a better adjunct to tai chi practice than running, which carries with it a far greater risk of injury. Swimming works all major muscle groups, provides great aerobic benefit, and nicely relieves the isometric compression of tai chi stances, especially when we remember to consciously lengthen our arms and legs during every stroke.

Cycling matches tai chi movements especially well because the circling movements of pedaling bear a relationship to the way we players use our hips. More, it works the leg muscles in complementary fashion. In particular, cycling builds the most lateral (outside) heads of the quadriceps (thigh muscles), whereas tai chi builds the medial (inside) heads. The combination makes for exceptionally well-toned legs. Unfortunately, performance "racing" bicycles designed for speed typically put the rider in a crouch, pressuring the perineum, wrists, elbows, and neck in an unhealthy fashion, and discouraging the straight spine and relaxed, open, upright posture tai chi requires. Instead, we may wish to opt either for an upright "cruiser" style bike, or a recumbent machine (there are some excellent recumbent tricycles available) that allows the cyclist to recline in a relaxed fashion.

In a 1997 magazine interview with tai chi Grandmaster Chen Quanzhong, I specifically asked him about cross-training. His answer, in characteristically abstruse fashion, was, "Cross-training is wonderful. It is very important. Don't do it." It took me quite a few more questions to divine that what he was trying to tell me was that there is very often a conflict between the way tai chi trains the body (coordinating muscles, sinking relaxing, spiraling) and what is required by other activities and sports. Once our bodies have really internalized the tai chi way of doing things and are able to apply it to any task, then cross-training can be very helpful. Until that time, it is better to avoid it. He emphasized that what he was really talking about was weightlifting.

That is because most weight lifting machines and exercises are designed for bodybuilders. As such, they emphasize muscular isolation. Isolating muscles makes them grow faster, and allows the bodybuilder to precisely sculpt his body. Isolation means disintegration, so sculpting is more about how a body looks than how it works. Since tai chi is all about function and integration, it is best to stay away from traditional, popular weight routines until "tai chi intelligence" has really saturated the mind and body. At that time, we can use kettle bells and dumbbells the way we might use heavy tai chi weapons, namely in integrated fashion, using the whole body to spiral, lift, turn, and move. In that way we obey tai chi principles, condition our ligaments and tendons, and have a good option where and when traditional weapons are not available.

There is also a product called the Bodyblade™, which uses vibration to train muscles and is especially useful training the explosive martial power known as tai chi Fajing. While this is an advanced technique, experienced players will find the Bodyblade™ a good adjunct to tai chi training right from the start, as it encourages relaxation and integration of body movements, and yet still tones and strengthens extremities and core.

Inflatable exercise balls are also fun cross-training tools for tai chi, and are especially useful in training our balance and strengthening our core. More, because many tai chi postures have us softening and closing the chest while we sink into the lower back, it is a healthy practice to lie backward over an exercise ball, arms outstretched to the side, and deeply and powerfully open the chest.

When it comes to clothing and accessories, any loose, comfortable clothing will suffice for practice, although the tai chi player will want to keep his or her core and extremities warm when training outside. There are quite a few suppliers that manufacture either martial arts gear that works well, or fashion items for tai chi demonstrations and those special occasions when you want to broadcast your passion.

Because tai chi requires a close relationship between the foot and the ground, and the ability to "grasp" the ground with the toes, choosing the right shoe makes a big difference to our practice. From the point of Traditional Chinese Medicine, thickly cushioned shoes not only make us unstable in our practice, they inhibit the compression of blood and lymph that takes place during normal walking—an important aid to circulation. Happily, the athletic shoe industry seems to have recently engaged a parallel concern, namely that the over-constructed shoes they have been building to cushion the joints from the shock of running actually weaken the muscles of the leg and foot by depriving them of their normal action. Returning to their roots, these companies are now offering lighter, simpler, thinner, more flexible running shoes, particularly those designed for barefoot use. These are quite good for tai chi, as are specialty martial arts shoes, thin-soled boat shoes, and kung fu slippers.

Many people like to practice tai chi to music using either a boom box or personal music player. The right music selection is important. Too slow and our tunes may dull us, too fast-paced and we will be unlikely to relax, too lyrical or melodic and our mind may follow the tune and deprive us of mindful awareness. Remember, our music should enhance the tai chi experience, not distract us from it.

MASTERY

There is one last element of tai chi practice that we have not discussed, and that is the emotional, philosophical, and spiritual benefits of mastery. Mastery itself seems almost to be a quaint concept these days, a term from another era, and certainly a quality supported by neither our culture nor our times. Information now develops at such a rate that whatever we learn in school is obsolete by the time we get out, and the skill set we develop at one job is unlikely to transfer to the next. The complexity of modern life has us more distracted than ever, and inundated by stimuli and messages that vie for our time in such a way that no one activity is likely to get much of it.

Few of us have or take the time to really focus. Indeed, the very notion of sticking with a single idea or skill or enterprise is under attack, if not directly then through the various vehicles of distraction that are available to us at all hours. This is a pity, because without narrow focus, long practice and plenty of patience we may occasionally be able to notice the patterns on the surface of life, but we will miss any revelation of its depths. There are layers upon layers to experience, and universes within worlds. Spending time at one thing long enough to truly command it develops deep awareness within us, lending us the ability to find truths that are all pervasive, meaningful and useful. The act of mastering something—anything—lends us self-knowledge, and in the process allows us to see past the differences in the world and substitute discernment for judgment.

Our tai chi practice offers us a chance to become masters of something that will stay with us for the rest of our lives. In no more time than we might spend watching television or surfing the Web, it offers us something nobody can ever take away from us, something classical, traditional, authentic, and of enduring value. Mastering tai chi does not merely mean controlling stress, defending our self, sharpening our mind, deepening our spirit, banishing illness, pushing back limitations, and prolonging youth. Mastering tai chi means mastering life. That is what makes it the perfect exercise.

Levels in Traditional Chen Style Tai Chi

BECAUSE THE CHEN FAMILY STYLE IS THE ORIGINAL FORM OF tai chi, a look at the traditional Chen curriculum helps to understand the way our mindbody can develop in all styles. Levels are based on the interaction between yin and yang (the opposing forces that Taoists believe exist in the world) in the body, which is to say between relaxation and tension, hardness and softness, concept and form, movement and stillness.

The goal of training is to harmonize these opposites. To understand how much yin or yang we are expressing in our body, the Chen curriculum uses a scale of ten. In the modern, Western world, most people begin with one level of yin and nine levels of yang. Once we have two yin and eight yang, it means we can turn the waist, but without connecting it to the rest of the body. Once we have three yin and seven yang, we can relax and sink with correct body mechanics, but we are still stiff. Once we have achieved four yin, we are good tai chi players. Once we have achieved five yin, we are in perfect balance.

LEVEL ONE – INTERNAL WORK COMMENCES

There are four degrees within this level. In the first, we learn about the concept of wuji and also learn to warm up our joints. In the second we learn to pay attention to shifting weight and we learn various tai chi stances. In the third we learn solo exercises and to sink the qi by relaxing, as well as starting rudimentary Pushing Hands. In the last level we learn the link between Lao Tzu's *Tao Te Ching* and tai chi practice. We also finish learning the first open-hand tai chi form and practice it approximately 1000 times with large, clear, relaxed movements and a straight back.

LEVEL TWO – ADVANCED PRACTICE BEGINS

Throughout the three degrees of this level the focus is on releasing tension and limitations of movement in the four major joints—the hips and the shoulders. In addition to specific exercises aimed at the hips and shoulders, we learn the straight sword (jian) form in this level, and to perform and counter basic joint locking (qinna). At the completion of this level, one must be able to handle a simple lock or grab applied inexpertly and the shoulders and hips have significantly opened.

LEVEL THREE – EXPERT WORK

All three degrees of this level emphasize pure relaxation. This is a very difficult level to complete, as it requires repeated and precise correction. Chen family tradition holds that few people reach this level in a lifetime of study, and even fewer leave it. We learn the single tai chi broadsword Dan Dao here, and our sensitivity in Pushing Hands makes the skills of that game quite practical. Upon completion of this level, we must be able to conduct to the ground any straight-line force equivalent to 150% of our body weight so long as that force is applied along the major direction of our stance.

LEVEL FOUR – PROFESSIONAL ACHIEVEMENT

This level focuses on mastering the tai chi-specific moving of the hips and body core we call Dantian rotation. This requires profound, functional relaxation. At this level, we learn the Spring and Autumn Broadsword Guan Dao and spear (qiang), as well as the explosive, second, open-hand routine known as Cannon Fist (Pao Cui). At this level, most other qinna practitioners cannot lock you, because your body will find an instinctive counter without thinking. Completing Level Three means you can handle another's strong force. Completing this level means they cannot handle yours.

LEVEL FIVE – MASTER

This level raises the strength and subtlety of the movements of the body's core and hips, the Dantian. At this level, long staff, Shi San Gan training is done, and a great deal of emphasis is put on meditation and other specialized internal work.

LEVELS SIX THROUGH TEN – ESOTERIC TEACHINGS

These are the levels during which mental, philosophical, and spiritual study rises to the fore. There are very few practitioners at these levels in China anymore, and even fewer in the West.

The Tai Chi Life

SOMETIMES WE EMBARK ON THE TAI CHI PATH BECAUSE IT fascinates us. Perhaps we are inspired by players practicing their flowing movements amidst morning doves and pine needles and ground fog at sunrise. Perhaps we envy the gracefulness we see when we watch tai chi, or the sudden explosions of power. Perhaps, without realizing the countless repetitions required, or the years of discipline and sore muscles, we somehow sense the joy in the practice and yearn to feel it.

Perhaps, too, we come to tai chi because the river of life seems to be sweeping us onto the rocks. If we have not been present or attended to our physical, mental, and spiritual health, we may feel the weight of all the choices we have wittingly or unwittingly made and come to tai chi to "fix" things. Disconnected from any sense of succor or source, we need tai chi to help easer our pain, anxiety, depression, or disease.

So we dive in. Almost immediately, we become aware of the distance between where we are in the art and where we would like to be. Suddenly, everyone in the world who has supernatural athletic talent seems to have congregated at tai chi class, while we seem not to be able to remember which of our feet is the left one. Our growing frustration is fed by the fact that we come from a culture that trains us to expect immediate gratification. After all, in our media-driven world, the American dream is more about sudden luck than good choices and careful planning, more about talent than trying.

Developing a relationship with tai chi may require us to maneuver counter to mainstream culture, to look for deep meaning, focus our attention, quiet our mind, and even to make a leap of faith—at least for the first year or so—and believe that there is a good reason why so many people find benefit in the art. Some time will have to pass before we can notice that our conflict resolution skills are better, that our fuse is longer and burns less hot, and that our legs respond more readily to stretching. We will have to practice for a while before we experience seemingly miraculous "saves" when we trip over a toy, or realize that our seemingly permanently sore back no longer hurts.

Too, we will have to contend with Chinese names, go to class when it's cold and we're tired, squash our self-doubt, learn martial etiquette, and even fake it sometimes. We will have to grasp the personal dynamics of our class and meet the challenge of the movements themselves before our digestion improves, before our allergies subside, before we can breathe easily through that sprint for the commuter train, before we can face our angry boss without a lump in our throat.

Of course, we can no more commit to tai chi after a couple of classes than we can realistically commit to a lover after a few dates. Like any other relationship, the benefits must become apparent before the love can flow, before the sacrifices come willingly, before the difficulties can be surmounted. Faith in the art and the words of the teacher are useful—even necessary—at the very outset, but at some point we have to dig deep and remind ourselves that we started all this because we believe the tai chi life to be a good one.

The good news is that it really is.

NOTES

INTRODUCTION

1. http://www.ncbi.nlm.nih.gov/pubmed/19554743

CHAPTER 5

1. http://theamt.com/oetzi_the_tyrolean_iceman_european_acupuncture_2000_years_before_china.htm

CHAPTER 7

1. http://www.ncbi.nlm.nih.gov/pubmed/22719790
2. http://www.ncbi.nlm.nih.gov/pubmed/17397428
3. http://www.ncbi.nlm.nih.gov/pubmed/22682857
4. http://www.ncbi.nlm.nih.gov/pubmed/22289280
5. http://www.ncbi.nlm.nih.gov/pubmed/22242736
6. http://www.ncbi.nlm.nih.gov/pubmed/22110979
7. http://www.ncbi.nlm.nih.gov/pubmed/22034119
8. http://www.ncbi.nlm.nih.gov/pubmed/21934474
9. http://www.ncbi.nlm.nih.gov/pubmed/21696487
10. http://www.ncbi.nlm.nih.gov/pubmed/21296261
11. http://www.ncbi.nlm.nih.gov/pubmed/21220083
12. http://www.ncbi.nlm.nih.gov/pubmed/19385493
13. http://www.ncbi.nlm.nih.gov/pubmed/19211957
14. http://www.ncbi.nlm.nih.gov/pubmed/18652095
15. http://www.ncbi.nlm.nih.gov/pubmed/18401235
16. http://www.ncbi.nlm.nih.gov/pubmed/18487902

17. http://www.ncbi.nlm.nih.gov/pubmed/18327432
18. http://www.ncbi.nlm.nih.gov/pubmed/17342248
19. http://www.ncbi.nlm.nih.gov/pubmed/11552205
20. http://www.ncbi.nlm.nih.gov/pubmed/7594155
21. http://www.ncbi.nlm.nih.gov/pubmed/7183208
22. http://www.ncbi.nlm.nih.gov/pubmed/22790795
23. http://www.ncbi.nlm.nih.gov/pubmed/20920810
24. http://www.ncbi.nlm.nih.gov/pubmed/22969831
25. http://www.ncbi.nlm.nih.gov/pubmed/21982141
26. http://www.ncbi.nlm.nih.gov/pubmed/22937260
27. http://www.ncbi.nlm.nih.gov/pubmed/22778122
28. http://www.ncbi.nlm.nih.gov/pubmed/22748753
29. http://www.ncbi.nlm.nih.gov/pubmed/22531145
30. http://www.ncbi.nlm.nih.gov/pubmed/22518287
31. http://www.ncbi.nlm.nih.gov/pubmed/18311126
32. http://www.ncbi.nlm.nih.gov/pubmed/21716708
33. http://www.ncbi.nlm.nih.gov/pubmed/21385664
34. http://www.ncbi.nlm.nih.gov/pubmed/22398352
35. http://www.ncbi.nlm.nih.gov/pubmed/20876465
36. http://www.ncbi.nlm.nih.gov/pubmed/20670413
37. http://www.ncbi.nlm.nih.gov/pubmed/19735238
38. http://www.ncbi.nlm.nih.gov/pubmed/17451612
39. http://www.ncbi.nlm.nih.gov/pubmed/16685074
40. http://www.ncbi.nlm.nih.gov/pubmed/6764710
41. http://www.ncbi.nlm.nih.gov/pubmed/6990211
42. http://www.ncbi.nlm.nih.gov/pubmed/6763007
43. http://www.ncbi.nlm.nih.gov/pubmed/16272874

BIBLIOGRAPHY

Aitken, Robert, with Kwok, Daniel W.Y., *Vegetable Roots Discourse— Wisdom from Ming China on Life and Living*, USA, Shoemaker Hoard, 2006

Ames, Roger T. and Hall, David, L., *Dao De Jing*, New York, Ballantine Books, 2003

Belyea, Charles, and Tainer, Steven, *Dragon's Play—A New Taoist Transmission of the Complete Experience of Human Life,* Berkeley, California, Great Circle Lifeworks, 1991

Bisio, Tom, *A Tooth from the Tiger's Mouth*, New York, Simon & Schuster, 2004

Boldt, Laurence, *The Tao of Abundance*, New York, Penguin, 1999

Breslow, Arieh Lev, *Beyond the Closed Door*, Jerusalem, Israel, Almond Blossom Press, 1995

Byrne, Patrick M. *Tao Te Ching*, Garden City Park, New York, Square One Publishers, 2002

Capra, Fritjof, *The Tao of Physics*, Boston, Massachusetts, Shambhala, 1991

Carolan, Trevor, *Return To Stillness—Twenty-Five Years With A Tai Chi Master,* New York, Marlowe and Company, 2003

Chang, Jolan, *The Tao of Love and Sex,* New York, E.P. Dutton, 1977

Chen, Mark, *Old Frame Chen Family Taijiquan,* Berkeley, California, North Atlantic Books, 2004

Chuckrow, Robert, *The Tai Chi Book*, Boston, Massachusetts, YMAA Publication Center, 1998

Chung, Tsai Chih, *Zhuangzi Speaks—The Music of Nature*, Princeton, NJ, Princeton University Press, 1992

Cleary, Thomas, *The Taoist Classics* vols. 1–4, Boston, Shambhala, 2003

Cleary, Thomas, *Thunder in the Sky*, Boston, Massachusetts, Shambhala, 1993

Cleary, Thomas, *The Way of the World*, Boston, Massachusetts, Shambhala, 2009

Cooper, J.C., *Taoism—The Way of the Mystic*, New York, Samuel Weiser, 1972

Cousineau, Phil, *Once and Future Myths*, Berkeley, California, Conari Press, 2001

Cuevas, Antonio (editor), *Martial Arts Are Not Just for Kicking Butt*, Berkeley, California, North Atlantic Books, 1998

Dang, Tri Thong, *Beyond the Known*, Rutland, Vermont, Charels E. Tuttle Company, 1993

David, Catherine, *The Beauty of Gesture—The Invisible Keyboard of Piano & T'ai Chi*, Berkeley, California, North Atlantic Books, 1996

Davis, Barbara, *The Taijiquan Classics—An Annotated Translation*, Berkeley, California, Blue Snake Books, 2004

Delza, Sophia, *The T'ai—Chi Ch'uan Experience*, Albany, New York, State University of New York Press, 1996

Deng, Ming-Dao, *Scholar Warrior—An Introduction to the Tao in Everyday Life*, New York, NY, HarperCollins, 1990

Diepersloot, Jan, *Warriors of Stillness—Meditative Traditions in the Chinese Martial Arts*, vols. 1&2, Walnut Creek, California, Center For Healing and the Arts, 1995

Drageter, Donn F., and Smith, Robert W., *Comprehensive Asian Fighting Arts*, Tokyo, Kodansha, 1969

Dreher, Diane, *The Tao of Inner Peace*, New York, HarperCollins, 1990

Eisenberg David (with Wright, Thomas Lee) *Encounters with Qi*, New York, Penguin Books, 1987

Emerson, Margaret, *Breathing Underwater*, Berkeley, California, North Atlantic Books, 1993

Fields, Rick, *The Code of the Warrior*, New York, HarperCollins, 1991

Frantzis, B.K., *The Power of Internal Martial Arts*, Berkeley, California, North Atlantic Books, 1998

Gallagher, Winfred, *Spiritual Genius*, New York, NY, Random House, 2002

Gilligan, Peter, *What Is Tai Chi*, London, Singing Dragon Press, 2010

Gilman, Michael, *A String of Pearls*, Port Townsend, Washington, Turning Point Press, 1996

Goleman, Daniel, et al., *Measuring the Immeasurable*, Boulder, Colorado, Sounds True, Inc. 2008

Grossman, Richard, *The Tao of Emerson*, New York, New York, Modern Library, 2007

Hamill, Sam, *Tao Te Ching*, Boston, Massachusetts, Shambhala, 2005

Heckler, Richard Strozzi, *In Search of the Warrior Spirit*, Berkeley, California, North Atlantic Books, 1990

Hoff, Benjamin, *The Tao of Pooh*, New York, Dutton, 1981

Hoff, Benjamin, *The Te of Piglet*, New York, Penguin, 1992

Horwood, Graham, *Tai Chi Chuan and the Code Of Life*, London, Singing Dragon, 2008

Hsun Tzu, *Basic Writings*, Burton Watson trans., New York, Columbia University Press, 1963

Huang, Chungliang Al, *Embrace Tiger, Return to Mountain*, Berkeley, California, Celestial Arts, 1973

Huang, Jane, *The Primordial Breath*, vol.2. Torrance, California, Original Books, 1990

Huang, Tao, Master, *Laoism—The Complete Teachings of Lao Zi*, Atlanta, Georgia, Humanics Trade Group, 2000

Hyams, Joe, *Zen in the Martial Arts*, Los Angeles, California, J.P. Tarcher Inc., 1979

James, Andy, *The Spiritual Legacy of the Shaolin Temple*, Essex, England, Wisdom Publications, 2005

Jou, Tsung Hwa, *The Tao of Tai—Chi Chuan—Way to Rejuvenation*, Warwick New York, Tai Chi Foundation, 1981

Kauz, Herman, *Push-Hands*, Woodstock, New York, The Overlook Press, 1997

Kauz, Herman, *The Martial Spirit*, Woodstock, New York, The Overlook Press, 1977

Kohn, Livia, *The Taoist Experience*, New York, State University of New York Press, 1993

Lash, John, *The Spirit of Tai Chi*, London, Vega Books, 2002

Lash, John, *The Yin of Tai Chi*, London, Vega Books, 2002

Leekley, Guy, *Tao Te Ching*, The Woodlands, Texas, Anusara Books 2004

Levy, Howard S. and Ishihara, Akira, *The Tao Of Sex*, Lower Lake, California, Integral Publishing, 1968

Liang, Shou-Yu and Wu, Wen-Ching, *Qigong Empowerment*, Rhode Island, The Way of the Dragon Publishing, 1997

Little, Stephen, *Taoism And The Arts Of China*, Chicago, Illinois, The Art Institute of Chicago, 2000

Liu, Da, *T'ai Chi Ch'uan and Meditation*, New York, Schocken Books, 1986

Liu, Da, *The Tao of Health and Longevity*, New York, Paragon House, 1991

Liu, Tianjun, et al., *Chinese Medical Qigong*, Philadelphia, Pennsylvania, Singing Dragon, 2010

Lowenthal, Wolfe, *Gateway to the Miraculous*, Berkeley, California, Frog Ltd., 1994

Lu, K'uan Yu, *The Secrets of Chinese Meditation*, York Beach, Maine, Samuel Weiser, 1964

Lu, K'uan Yu, *Taoist Yoga*, San Francisco, California, Weiser Books, 1973

Lutang, Sun, *A Study of Taijiquan*, Tim Cartmell, trans., Berkeley, California, North Atlantic Books, 2003

Mair, Victor, *Tao Te Ching*, New York, Quality Paperback Book Club, 1990

Man-ch'ing, Cheng, and Smith, Robert, *Tai Chi—The "Supreme Ultimate" Exercise For Health, Sport, And Self-Defense*, Rutland, Vermont, Charles Tuttle Co. 1967

Miszewski, Michael, *Spiritual Dimensions of the Martial Arts*, Rutland, Vermont, Charles E. Tuttle Co., 1996

Mitchell, Stephen, *Tao Te Ching*, New York, Harper & Row, 1988

Nan, Huai-Chin, *Tao & Longevity—Mind-Body Transformation*, translated by Chu, Wen Kuan, York Beach, Maine, Samuel Weiser, 1984

O'Brien, Jess, *Nei Jia Quan—Internal Martial Arts*, 2nd edition, Berkeley, California, Blue Snake Books, 2007

Osho, *Tao—The Pathless Path*, New York, Columbia University Press, 2002

Porter, Bill (Red Pine) *Taoteching*, San Francisco, California, Mercury House, 1996

Roberts, Holly, *Tao Te Ching*, Anjeli Press, USA, 2005

Roberts, Moss, *Tao Te Ching*, Berkeley and Los Angeles, California, University of California Press, 2001

Rosenbaum, Michael, *The Fighting Arts*, Boston, Massachusetts, YMAA Publication Center, 2002

Russell, Stephen, *Barefoot Doctor's Guide To The Tao*, New York, Times Books, 1998

Shing, Yen-Ling, *Chen Style T'ai Chi Ch'uan*, Tokyo, Japan, Sugawara Martial Arts Institute, 1993

Silberstorff, Jan, *Chen—Living Taijiquan in the Classical Style*, London, Singing Dragon, 2003

Sim, Davidine Siaw-Voon and Gaffney, *Chen Style Taijiquan – The Source Of Chinese Boxing*, Berkeley, California, North Atlantic Books, 2002

Simpkins, C. Alexander and Annellen, M., *Simple Taoism—A Guide to Living in Balance,* Vermont, Tuttle, 1999

Soeng, Mu, *Trust In Mind—The Rebellion of Chinese Zen,* Essex, England, Wisdom Publications, 2004

Soho, Takuan, *The Unfettered Mind*, William Scott Wilson, trans., New York, Kodansha, 1986

Starr, Jonathan, *Tao Te Ching*, New York, NY, Jeremy P. Tarcher/Putnam, 2001

Talbot, Michael, *The Holographic Universe*, New York, NY, HarperCollins, 1991

Tcherne, Oleg, *Alchemy of Pushing Hands*, London, Singing Dragon, 2004

Waley, Arthur, *The Way and Its Power*, New York, Grove Press, 1958

Walker, Brian Browne, *Hua Hu Ching—The Unknown Teachings of Lao Tzu,* New York, HarperCollins, 1992

Watts, Alan, and Watts, Mark, *Taoism—Way Beyond Seeing—The Edited Transcripts*, Tokyo, Japan, Charles Tuttle & Co. 1997

Watts, Alan, *Does It Matter*, Novato, California, New World Library, 2007

Watts, Alan, *Eastern Wisdom, Modern Life*, Novato, California, New World Library, 1994

Watts, Alan, *The Book*, New York, Random House, 1966

Watts, Alan, *This Is It*, New York, Random House, 1958

Watts, Alan, *Cloud-Hidden, Whereabouts Unknown*, New York, Random House, 1968

Wile, Douglas, *Lost Tai-Chi Classics from the Late Ch'ing Dynasty*, Albany, New York, State University of New York Press, 1996

Wilson, William Scott, *Lao Tzu—Tao Te Ching*, Japan, Kodansha 2010

Wing, R.L. *The Tao Of Power*, New York, Broadway Books, 1986

Wiseman, Nigel, Ye, Feng, *A Practical Dictionary Of Chinese Medicine*, Brookline, Massachusetts, Paradigm Publications, 1998

Wong, Eva, *Cultivating Stillness*, Boston, Massachusetts, Shambhala, 1992

Wong, Eva, *Lieh-Tzu, A Taoist Guide to Practical Living*, Boston, Massachusetts, Shambhala Publications, 1995

Xi'an, Wang, *Chen Family Taijiquan Tuishou*, Naroubra, NSW, Australia, INBI Matrix PTY LTD, 2009

Xin, Chen, *The Illustrated Canon Of Chen Family Taijiquan*, Maroubra, NSW, Australia, INBI Matrix PTY LTD, 2007

Yang, Jwing—Ming, *Taijiquan Theory*, Boston, Massachusetts, YMAA Publication Center, 2003

Yang, Yang, *Taijiquan – The Art of Nurturing, The Science of Power*, Champaign, Illinois, Zhenwu Publications, 2005

Yasuo, Yuasa, *The Body, Self-Cultivation, And Ki-Energy*, Albany, New York, State University of New York Press, 1993

Yun, Zhang, *The Art Of Chinese Swordsmanship—A Manual of Taiji Jian*, Boston, Massachusetts, Shambhala, 1998

Yun, Zhang, *The Complete Taiji Dao—The Art of Chinese Saber*, Berkeley, California, Blue Snake Books, 2009

Yutang, Lin, *The Importance of Living*, New York, NY, HarperCollins, 1937

Zhang, Yu Huan, and Rose, Ken, *A Brief History of Qi*, Brookline, Massachusetts, Paradigm Publications, 2001.

ARTHUR ROSENFELD,
AUTHOR AND TAI CHI MASTER

Arthur Rosenfeld began his formal martial arts training in 1980 and has studied deeply in China and the United States. A Yale graduate, he did graduate work at Cornell and the University of California, has his needle in the vein of Chinese tai chi grandmasters, and is dedicated to personal transformation and social change through the application of Taoist philosophy and movement. In 2012 the Chinese government honored him by ordaining him a Taoist monk at the Chun Yang (Pure Yang) Taoist Temple in Guangzhou, the first Westerner to be so honored. He was named Tai Chi Master of The Year at the World Congress on Qigong and Traditional Chinese Medicine in 2011, and received the Action On Film Festival's Maverick Award for excellence in martial arts in the media in August 2012.

Rosenfeld hosts the hit national PBS show *Longevity Tai Chi with Arthur Rosenfeld*, contributes to such magazines as *Vogue*, *Vanity Fair*, and *Parade*, and has been cited in numerous national magazines. Rosenfeld blogs on *The Huffington Post*, and his offerings also appear in *The Wall Street Journal*, *Fox Business News*, and numerous other websites and newspapers nationwide.

Rosenfeld has penned thirteen critically acclaimed books, some of which have sold bestseller numbers and been optioned to Hollywood. Along with the Dalai Lama, he was a finalist for the prestigious Books for a Better Life award for his bestseller *The Truth About Chronic Pain* (New York: Basic Books, 2003), and his prize-winning novels have recently featured Chinese philosophy and martial arts action. He holds corporate and open workshops internationally and around the country, and teaches beginning and advanced tai chi students at his home base in South Florida.

Visit Arthur's Website: www.arthurrosenfeld.com
Email Arthur: arthur@arthurrosenfeld.com

INDEX

G

Gall Bladder Meridian, 103
Genes, 141
Governing (Du) Vessels, 100–101
Gravity, 41–42
Greater and Lesser Heavenly
    Circles, 100–101, 150–151,
    154–160
Greater Heavenly Circle, 150–151,
    157–160
Green Dragon Extends its Claws
    (Qing Long Xian Zhua), 176
Green movement, 39
Guan Dao (Spring and Autumn
    Broadsword), 174–175, 213
Guan Yu, 174
Gyros, 60–61

H

Habit, 61–62
Halberd (Spring and Autumn
    Broadsword, Guan Do),
    174–175, 213
Hao Wei Chen, 205
Harvard Women's Health Watch,
    8
Health
    balanced, 140–142
    chronic issues, 27, 58
    lifestyle diseases, 81
    sciatica, 63
    stress and, 10
    See also Medicine
Heart Meridian, 102
Heavenly Circles, 100–101,
    150–151, 154–160
Holy Ghost, 97

Homeostasis. *See* Wuji
Honored father (Sifu), 195
Honored uncle (Sifu), 195
Ho'o, Marshall, 166
Hsing-I Ch'uan (Mind Boxing),
    205
Hui Yin (Merging Perineum), 32

I

I-Ching, Book of Changes
    (Yiqing), 53, 74, 167
Information, overload of, 36–37,
    210
Integrative Medicine, 139, 140
Internal arts, 5–6
Intuition, 191
Iron Bull Plows the Field (Tie Niu
    Geng Di), 176
Iron lollipop, 21–22

J

Jedis, 2
Ji, 66
Jian (double-edged sword, short
    metal cudgels), 170–172, 176,
    212
Jian Jing (Shoulder Well), 32, 161,
    162
Jiang Fa, 204
Jin Bu (advance), 193
Jing (sexual fluid essence), 106,
    128–129
Joint locking (qinna), 168, 212

K

Karate-do (way of the empty
    hand), 74

Ki, 97
Kidney Meridian, 103
Knife (Dao), 172–173, 174
Kung fu, 3–5
Kung Fu (television series), xiv

L

Lao Ghong, 162
Lao Tzu, 3, 53, 136
 on discipline, 110
 on effortlessness, 16
 as mythical, 74–75
 surname of, 54–55
Large Intestine Meridian, 101
Learning
 in brain, 62
 tai chi, 197–202
Lee, Bruce, xiv, 3, 140, 186
Lesser Heavenly Circle, 150–151,
 154–156
Levels, 13, 211–213
Li (strength), 26
Li Xin, 54
Li Xiyue, 54
Li Zhong, 54
Lieh (change direction), 193
Lieh Tzu, 74
Life Gate (Ming Men), 32, 158,
 162, 163
Lifestyle diseases, 81
Lineage, 43–44, 202
Listening, 124
Liu (Roll-back), 66, 193
Liver Meridian, 103
Long wooden pole (Da Gan),
 176–177

Lucas, George, 2
Lung Meridian, 101
Lymphatic system, 34

M

Maintain a central position
 (Zhong Ting), 193
Mamet, David, 200
Mana, 97
Mao Zedong, 53, 64
Marine Corps, U.S., 21
Martial arts
 in China, 5
 exchanges in, 185
 self-defense, 4, 178–184
 softness in, 6
 tai chi as, 63–64, 165–189
 watercourse, 185–187
 See also specific martial arts
Martial etiquette (wu de),
 195–197
Martial intention (yi), 25
Mastery, 195, 209–210
The Matrix (movie), 37
Medicine
 benefits of, 146–147
 bone-setting, 7, 8
 Integrative, 139, 140
 National Library of Medicine/
 National Institutes of Health,
 U.S., 141, 146
 See also Traditional Chinese
 Medicine
Meditation
 relaxation and, 161
 standing, 157–160